Out of Sight, Not Out of Mind

PERSONAL AND PROFESSIONAL PERSPECTIVES ON AGE-RELATED MACULAR DEGENERATION

Lindy Bergman
with The Chicago Lighthouse for People
Who Are Blind or Visually Impaired

Jennifer E. Miller, Esq., *Editor*

AFB PRESS
American Foundation for the Blind

Printed in the United States of America

Library of Congress Cataloging-in-Publication Data

Bergman, Lindy.
   Out of sight, not out of mind : personal and professional perspectives on age-related macular degeneration / Lindy Bergman with The Chicago Lighthouse for People Who Are Blind or Visually Impaired ; Jennifer E. Miller, editor. — Updated and expanded version.
      p. ; cm.
   Includes bibliographical references.
   ISBN 978-0-89128-485-7 (pbk. : alk. paper) — ISBN 978-0-89128-486-4 (ascii cd) — ISBN 978-0-89128-487-1 (e-book)
   I. Miller, Jennifer E. II. Chicago Lighthouse (Organization) III. American Foundation for the Blind. IV. Title.
   [DNLM: 1. Macular Degeneration—psychology. 2. Macular Degeneration—etiology. 3. Macular Degeneration—rehabilitation. WW 270]

   617.7'35—dc23
                            2011047591

This is an updated and expanded version of *Out of Sight, Not Out of Mind*, by Lindy Bergman, published in 1998 by The University of Chicago Hospitals.

The American Foundation for the Blind—the organization to which Helen Keller devoted her life—is a national nonprofit devoted to expanding the possibilities for people with vision loss.

It is the policy of the American Foundation for the Blind to use in the first printing of its books acid-free paper that meets the ANSI Z39.48 Standard. The infinity symbol that appears above indicates that the paper in this printing meets that standard.

Contents WITHDRAWN

Foreword

How We Choose To See It

Jonathan Safran Foer

——— ———

I was desperate to see them with my own eyes. And despite having given away the great majority of the art she's owned, Lindy Bergman still had a number of Joseph Cornell's most magical works in her Chicago apartment at that time.

"Why on earth would she invite me into her home?" I asked the museum curator who had suggested I be in touch with Lindy.

"Because she's Lindy Bergman, and that's what she's like."

I arrived an hour early, and walked nervous loops around her building. When the time came, the doorman led me to the elevator, the doors closed, and frankly, I had no idea what to expect. I didn't know what she looked like, what her apartment looked like, how it would feel to be in the presence of those objects I'd spent so much time thinking about. And she knew nothing about me, beyond my interest in Cornell. The elevator doors opened and we were

———

Jonathan Safran Foer is an award-winning author best known for his books *Everything Is Illuminated*, *Extremely Loud and Incredibly Close*, *Eating Animals*, and other works. He also has a great love of the artist Joseph Cornell.

both surprised: the art enthusiast she had invited over was only 17; the art collector I was coming to meet was effectively blind.

The appointment, which was supposed to last 15 minutes, went on for more than two hours. It was one of the most memorable afternoons of my life. She guided me from room to room of her beautiful apartment, describing, at length, artworks she couldn't, herself, see. And we talked: about our shared love for Cornell, of course, but also about our families, our pasts, and our hopes for the future. One hope we shared was that it would not be our last meeting. It wasn't. That afternoon was 15 years ago. Since then, Lindy and I have grown and maintained a friendship that is as dear to me as any I have.

There aren't enough pages in this book to hold all of the lessons I've learned from Lindy, but in a sense they all boil down to the same thing: determined optimism. We have very little control over what happens to us, but full control over how we choose to see it. I've been so lucky to see, with my own eyes, how Lindy has dealt with the loss of hers. Rather than object to the unfairness of it, or resign herself to a diminished existence, she has chosen to live. Her social calendar is literally as full as that of anyone I know, and she has a seemingly unlimited thirst for new experience, conversation, and friendship. She chooses to see life—with all of its difficulties—as a gift to spend every day opening. She's Lindy Bergman, and that's what she's like. And it's what we all should strive to be more like.

About the Contributors

ABOUT THE AUTHOR

Lindy Bergman is a supporter of art and health institutions in her home city of Chicago, Illinois, and sits on the boards of many philanthropic organizations. She helped establish the Bergman Institute for Psychological Support at The Chicago Lighthouse for People Who Are Blind or Visually Impaired. Her donated artworks form the Lindy and Edwin Bergman Collection of surrealist art at the Art Institute of Chicago. Mrs. Bergman published the original edition of *Out of Sight, Not Out of Mind* in 1998.

ABOUT THE EDITOR

Jennifer E. Miller, J.D., LL.M., is Director of Development for Individual and Planned Giving at The Chicago Lighthouse for People Who Are Blind or Visually Impaired. Prior to joining The Chicago Lighthouse, she was a practicing attorney and Clinical Assistant Professor of Law at Northwestern Law School in Chicago. She has over 11 years' experience teaching writing, literature, and law to college, community college, and law students. Miller also holds master's degrees in English and taxation law.

ABOUT THE CONTRIBUTORS

Kara Crumbliss, O.D., is Director of Clinical Services and a low vision optometrist at The Chicago Lighthouse for People Who Are Blind or Visually Impaired. In addition, she serves as Clinical Assistant Professor of Optometry and Low Vision Rehabilitation and Ocular Disease Residency Coordinator at the Illinois College of Optometry in Chicago and Adjunct Clinical Professor of Optometry with the University of Missouri, St. Louis. Her research interests include the association of low vision with Charles Bonnet Syndrome, cognitive impairment, and Alzheimer's disease. She has authored journal articles and lectured extensively on these and other topics related to low vision rehabilitation.

Gerald Allen Fishman, M.D., is Director of the Pangere Center for Hereditary Retinal Diseases at The Chicago Lighthouse for People Who Are Blind or Visually Impaired. He is also Adjunct Professor in the Department of Ophthalmology and Visual Sciences at the University of Illinois at Chicago, where he previously held the Marion Schenk, Esq., Endowed Chair of Ophthalmology, and serves as chair of the clinical scientific advisory board of the Foundation Fighting Blindness. A world-renowned ophthalmologist, researcher, and academic specializing in inherited retinal diseases, Dr. Fishman has published over 340 papers in refereed journals, as well as book chapters and other publications, in addition to numerous lectures and presentations. His many honors include Best Doctors in America and Top Doctor in Chicago, the Beacon of Excellence Award from The Chicago Lighthouse, and Distinguished Faculty Award from the University of Illinois College of Medicine at Chicago.

Patricia Grant, M.S., is Director of the Low Vision Research Department at The Chicago Lighthouse for People Who Are Blind or Visually Impaired and Research Specialist, Department of Ophthalmology and Visual Sciences at the University of Illinois at Chicago. She has published several journal articles on macular degeneration and retinal dysfunction. Ms. Grant is currently a Ph.D. candidate in Community Health Sciences at the University of Illinois at Chicago School of Public Health.

Thomas B. Perski, M.A., is Senior Vice President of Rehabilitation Services at The Chicago Lighthouse for People Who Are Blind or Visually Impaired. He was previously the Director of Vision Services at Vision Care Ophthalmic Technologies in Saratoga, CA; Founder and Clinical Director of Southwest Low Vision in Tucson, Arizona; and Founder and Executive Director of Macular Degeneration International in Tucson. He has published several articles on low vision rehabilitation and given numerous professional presentations. Perski received the 2004 Margaret Blum Award as Professional Worker of the Year, from Arizona Association for Education and Rehabilitation of the Blind and Visually Impaired and the 1998 Bower Achievement Award in Recognition of Outstanding Support of Macular Degeneration Research at Wills Eye Hospital, Philadelphia.

David M. C. Rakofsky, Psy.D., is Associate Director of the Bergman Institute for Psychological Support at The Chicago Lighthouse for People Who Are Blind or Visually Impaired and a clinical psychologist in private practice as president of Wellington Counseling Group in Chicago and its surrounding suburbs. Prior to joining The Lighthouse to establish the psychological support program, he was a research consultant to the Low Vision Laboratory within the Department of Ophthalmology and Visual Sciences at University of Illinois at Chicago. Dr. Rakofsky has dedicated much of his previous practice to service within Chicago area community mental health centers and to the training of future psychologists.

Alfred A. Rosenbloom, Jr., O.D., D.O.S., who holds the Krumrey Chair in Low Vision at The Chicago Lighthouse for People Who Are Blind or Visually Impaired, is one of the founders of its Low Vision Rehabilitation Service. Dr. Rosenbloom was formerly Distinguished Professor at Illinois College of Optometry in Chicago and served as its dean and then president for over 25 years. He is also Clinical Professor in the Department of Ophthalmology at the University of Illinois Medical Center. Dr. Rosenbloom is author of numerous scientific papers and a contributing author to or editor of several textbooks, including the third edition of *Vision and Aging.* Dr. Rosenbloom has received lifetime achievement awards from The Chicago Lighthouse and Prevent Blindness America, as well as the Distinguished Service Award from the American Optometric Association where he served previously as acting chair of their Low Vision Rehabilitation and Geriatric Services; the 2007 Humanitarian of the Year award from Volunteer Optometric Services to Humanity, of which he is past president; the William Feinbloom Memorial Award for excellence in low vision services; and the Migel Medal from the American Foundation for the Blind.

Janet P. Szlyk, Ph.D., is President and Executive Director of The Chicago Lighthouse for People Who Are Blind or Visually Impaired. She is also Adjunct Professor in the

Departments of Ophthalmology and Visual Sciences, Bio-engineering, and Psychology at the University of Illinois at Chicago, where she previously served as Professor and Director of the Low Vision Research Laboratory in the Department of Ophthalmology and Visual Sciences and Professor in the Bioengineering and Psychology Departments. Dr. Szlyk is widely published in the field of vision rehabilitation and has served as principal investigator on numerous federally funded research projects. She regularly serves as a reviewer for journals and grants and as a consultant to the U.S. Food and Drug Administration. Dr. Szlyk received the Rehabilitation Research Career Scientist Award from the U.S. Department of Veterans Affairs' Rehabilitation Research and Development Service in 1999 and 2006.

PART 1

Personal Experiences

OUT OF SIGHT, NOT OUT OF MIND—LINDY BERGMAN'S STORY

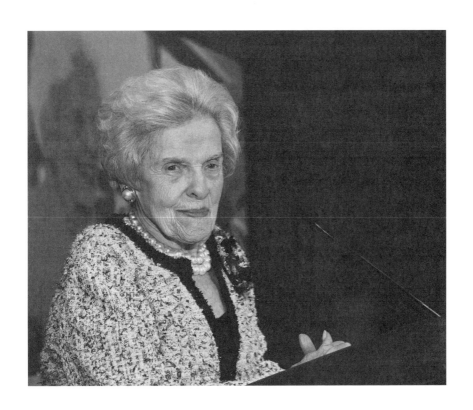

Preface

Lindy Bergman with Jennifer E. Miller

Despite the fact that she'd been diagnosed with age-related macular degeneration (AMD) three years before, Chicagoan Lindy Bergman decided to rejuvenate her garden when she was 77 years old. She had come to this decision after much thought, because her initial reaction to her diagnosis had been one of fear and dismay.

The vision in her left eye had decreased significantly due to the growth of new blood vessels and subsequent scarring in the retina, the signs of AMD. Lindy had experienced reduced depth perception and a loss of visual clarity. But after going through a process of adjustment, her lifelong optimism began to reassert itself.

Accordingly, that spring, Lindy planted a flower garden full of plants that would have bright colors that she could see. Lindy wanted a kaleidoscope of colors: red roses, blue delphiniums, orange daylilies, and purple clematis. She also wanted a butterfly bush to beckon the butterflies. The garden would take several seasons to establish itself, but Lindy knew that by the following summer, she would have vibrant strands of color that would change throughout the seasons.

Picture Lindy's garden in your mind. When the project was complete, that was all Lindy could do, too, because

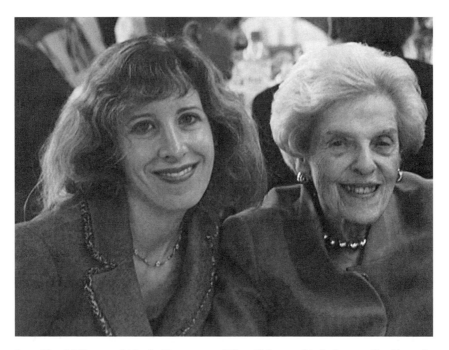

Jennifer Miller and Lindy Bergman (The Chicago Lighthouse for People Who Are Blind or Visually Impaired)

by then she truly felt the effects of macular degeneration. As the summer of that year commenced, so did the growth of new blood vessels in her good eye. The condition invaded her other eye and took the central vision there, as it had in her first eye. Now Lindy would know the full extent of vision loss associated with AMD. She could see only blurred groups of colors in her flower garden. She could no longer identify what flowers she was seeing, and she couldn't see the individual shapes of the flowers.

"This is very frustrating," Lindy sighed, mourning the disappearance of her sight. After a time, though, she realized that when she had first visualized the garden, she wasn't literally seeing it. She had pictured it before in her mind, and she could still do so.

"I haven't lost my garden," Lindy thought. "It may be out of sight, but it's not out of mind. And," she concluded, "neither am I! I may have lost my vision. However, that doesn't mean I have to lose my head, even though macular degeneration drives me crazy sometimes! I, too, may be out of sight, but I'm not out of mind!"

Lindy loved that garden. She added plants that filled the air with fragrances, and when her grandchildren described the fluttering butterflies, Lindy "saw" them, too.

OUT OF SIGHT NOW—STILL *NOT OUT OF MIND!*

Lindy first wrote those words over a decade ago. When she was originally diagnosed with macular degeneration nearly 20 years ago, she was the only one she knew who had this condition. Lindy had heard of the disease, but no one she knew personally was affected.

But, as the years passed, more and more people Lindy knew became diagnosed with AMD. She would often receive phone calls from peers, friends, and even people she didn't even know. They would see her at different functions around Chicago and were amazed. They all asked her the same questions: "How do you manage? How do you cope? How do you keep so optimistic?"

Lindy's thoughts became the foundation for the first part of this book, prose that she fashioned to help those experiencing AMD who are depressed and who are scared to lose their sight. To this day, Lindy still has people calling her with questions about how she copes.

Since Lindy's first wrote *Out of Sight, Not Out of Mind* in 1998, many changes have occurred. She sold her house with the garden, but she can still picture the garden in her mind. And she can still visualize her butterfly bush with the colorful insects flying around the bright flowers.

Another change that occurred was that Lindy decided it was time to update her book. Much research had been done on macular degeneration since then, and many new types of technology had become available to help those who have AMD regain their sense of independence. Lindy went to The Chicago Lighthouse for People Who Are Blind or Visually Impaired for assistance. It was not the first time Lindy had turned to The Lighthouse for help.

The Lighthouse's mission is to help people who are blind or visually impaired become independent and self-sufficient through its many programs and services. Located in Chicago, it has been helping individuals with visual impairments for over 100 years, and it is the largest social service agency in the Midwest. It also aids people all over the country through some of its national programs.

Lindy originally came to The Lighthouse for orientation and mobility training when she was first diagnosed with AMD. Over the years, she returned to The Lighthouse again and again for different services. She visited one of the optometrists at The Lighthouse's low vision clinic for an eye exam and for low vision care. She also frequented the adaptive technology center to see the latest developments in adaptive technology and to identify what could assist her in her own home. On her ophthalmologist's recommendation, she continued to consult with The Lighthouse staff and obtained a white cane as well as a talking thermometer. She also purchased a talking watch, which she still uses to this day. Finally, Lindy went to The Lighthouse for computer assistance, since the agency's computer staff are experts at helping people with low vision use computers.

When it came time to revise her book, it became clear that it was natural for Lindy to partner with The Lighthouse. It had helped her personally for so many years, and she knew about the quality of care it provided and the wonderful spirit of the people who work there. In addition, the low vision experts on staff could help Lindy augment her book and update it, and she viewed it as a place "that makes you feel really good to be there." This partnership resulted in Lindy's revised book, which you are reading right now.

TOOLS FOR READERS

The title *Out of Sight, Not Out of Mind: Personal and Professional Perspectives on Age-Related Macular Degeneration* reflects this book's focus on readers pursuing the topic of AMD and their needs. The first part of the book is written especially for people who have recently been diagnosed with AMD, who are asking the same questions Lindy often receives: "How do you manage? How do you cope? How do you keep so optimistic?" (In addition, the "Age-Related Macular Degeneration Guide," an appendix to this book, provides a handy summary of many of the facts about AMD and tips for living with this condition that are found throughout this volume.) It is hoped that *Out of Sight* will give such readers tools for coping with AMD and suggestions on successfully managing their lives with AMD. It is also hoped that, by its conclusion, they will "see" that even though a physical garden with butterflies may be out of sight, it isn't "out of mind," and they can still live highly successful and productive lives. We believe that professionals will also benefit from reading Lindy's story and her firsthand account, which provides perspective and insight into how their patients may experience AMD.

The second part of the book contains descriptions of some of the latest medical research on AMD and of current treatments and options for rehabilitation in low vision care. Drawing upon the experience of The Lighthouse's experts who focus on low vision services, it aims to show practitioners a model of comprehensive and effective services for helping patients and clients to cope with AMD in today's world. Professionals who work with people who are experiencing AMD—which may include ophthalmologists, optometrists, social workers, psychologists, and orientation and mobility specialists, among others—will find of wealth of information here, as will people experiencing AMD themselves and their families. Once readers with vision loss comprehend the various dimensions of AMD and the possible options for available services, they can better understand the alternatives for moving forward with their lives.

The book is intended to provide "tools for living." When someone is better equipped with the latest information, he or she may find it easier to know what to ask on the next visit to the ophthalmologist or optometrist, and to make informed decisions, leading to a more satisfying life.

So, read this book, and have hope. If you have any doubts about the possibilities, consider Lindy Bergman, a pioneer in the public discussion of AMD, who at the age of 93 is still living a successful and highly satisfying life.

CHAPTER 1

Gaining a Sense of AMD

The signs of age-related macular degeneration (AMD) are fairly straightforward: A doctor probably didn't need to tell you that you were having trouble seeing. What may not have been so clear, however, is exactly what it means to have AMD.

For me, I will never forget the day when I was at the beauty parlor, and I was looking at a poster. On impulse, just for a test, I tried seeing the difference between what I could see when I covered my left eye and then my right eye. When I covered my left eye and looked at the poster, I could see the poster of the latest hairstyle just fine. But I suddenly realized that when I covered my right eye, all I could see was a big blob. With this eye, what I should have been able to read was instead cloudy and murky. I was concerned, and understandably so!

When I got home, I immediately called my doctor, who wanted to see me right away. At my appointment, he called in a retina specialist, who quickly diagnosed my condition as age-related macular degeneration. (If you are concerned or wondering about your own vision, you can check it to make sure that it hasn't changed or monitor

A Simple Test: The Amsler Grid

One method doctors have to help you monitor your central eye condition is the Amsler Grid. Some changes can be gradual, so you may not notice them over a period of time. That is why it is so important to see your eye doctor regularly. And, if changes in your eyes are detected by your eye care professional, treatment can potentially help.

This simple test, called the Amsler Grid, can help you detect changes in your vision that you might not otherwise notice. This grid is a sheet of graph paper with a reference dot in the center similar to the one shown here, but bigger.

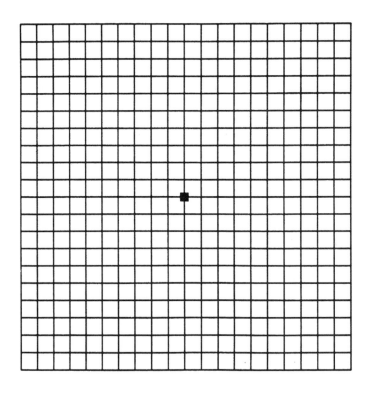

Here is how to use it:

+ Hold the grid 14 inches in front of you in a good light. Be sure to use your corrective glasses or reading glasses if you wear them normally.
+ Cover one eye.
+ Look directly at the center dot with your uncovered eye.
+ While looking at this dot, determine whether all of the lines of the grid appear straight and uninterrupted and have the same contrast.
+ Repeat these steps with the other eye.

If any part of the grid is missing or looks wavy, blurred, or dark, call your eye doctor immediately. (By the way, a good place to hang it is on your bathroom mirror, so you don't forget to do the test every day.)

it with your eye care specialist by using the technique described in "A Simple Test: The Amsler Grid.")

THE MACULAR DEGENERATION DIAGNOSIS

If you've received a diagnosis of macular degeneration, it may be helpful for you to know that you will probably never be completely blind if you have AMD alone. Seeing is based on two components: central vision and peripheral, or side, vision. Macular degeneration affects your central vision, blocking out what would be directly in front of you. Peripheral vision, in contrast, is the vision that occurs at the very outside of your direct viewing area as you face straight ahead. It is the part of vision that detects objects to the side. For example, peripheral vision tells you if a car is approaching from your left or right side. AMD may also leave your peripheral vision blurry. You may now see as if you were looking through a cloud or as though you're looking through a mist. But it is likely you will still be able to see shadows or make out images.

If your doctor hasn't talked to you about what you will still be able to see with macular degeneration, ask him or her about it. In fact, it can be helpful to make a list of all of your questions. Then ask your doctor about the specifics and have him or her tell you whatever you feel you need to know. You may be encouraged to know that macular degeneration is not like being in a windowless room with all the lights shut off. Your central vision will be affected, but usually, in approximately half the cases, AMD does not occur equally in both eyes. In other words, with macular degeneration, about 50 percent of the time, one eye generally sees better than the other.

You may find it important to keep in mind that there is a big difference between loss of vision and complete blindness. Most people, having been diagnosed with AMD, initially believe that they will become completely blind. I was told by a wonderful retinal ophthalmologist the very first day I was diagnosed with AMD that "with AMD, you will never be black-blind [and by that he meant completely blind]. You will always be able to manage." I never forgot these words, which have provided me great comfort, and they remain true nearly two decades later. Even though this eye doctor was very young, I believed him. I remember thinking at the time that he had an open and honest approach to the disease I now apparently had. These words have been my mantra for some time now. I think that if you, too, remember these words, they may help you and bring you a long way toward coping with AMD.

I have had many friends call me over the years after they have been diagnosed with AMD. Understandably, they are scared, shocked, anxious, and depressed after hearing this startling news. These are common feelings in reaction to this diagnosis, so if you are feeling the same way, that is to be expected and is completely normal. It may take time for you to completely digest the idea of having macular degeneration and to understand its consequences. But once you do, you may also begin to realize that you can still have the life that you would like to live, with some help from a few different places.

NOW IT IS TIME TO *LIVE* WITH MACULAR DEGENERATION

Macular degeneration is not like other more debilitating diseases. It may not completely incapacitate you. Indeed, when it affects just one eye, you will in all likelihood find that you can do a majority of the things you've always done. Your depth perception may be off, and your reflexes may be slower, but other than stubbing your toes more often than before, you may not notice a dramatic difference in your lifestyle.

If the disease begins to affect your second eye, then you may begin to have to compensate for a lack of vision. That is what happened to me. You may find that reading without the help of visual devices may become nearly impossible. Unfortunately, you eventually may have to give up driving. I didn't bemoan the loss of my driving when I was told to give it up, but I know that for others, it can be devastating. A fair number of my friends have had to give up driving, and it was extremely hard for them, when they were used to driving independently to the grocery store or other places.

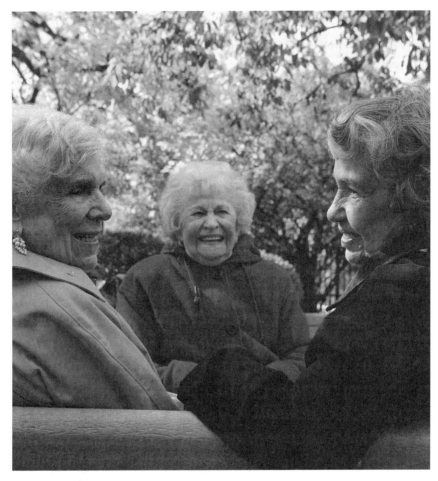

Losing vision doesn't mean having to retreat from the world. Spending time with family and friends helps prevent feeling isolated. (The Chicago Lighthouse for People Who Are Blind or Visually Impaired)

Overall, many of the activities you're accustomed to doing may become harder to accomplish on your own. However, there are many ways to accomplish those activities, and you will be able to learn them, just as I was. I have included some tips in the following chapters, which I hope will help.

Also, the human spirit is resilient. You may find that on some days, you think you can see more than you could the day before. Maybe getting around is not as frightening as it seemed to be at first. You may find that the more you try to do, the more you actually can do.

This is because you are gradually adapting. After a while it may not feel so strange to continue to use phrases such as "I see," or "the way I look at it." You'll also learn to set the lights in your home at a level that helps you define shapes and images more easily. And you'll learn to move your eyes so that you can position objects within your peripheral vision, rather than trying to make them out entirely in your central vision, especially if you obtain low vision services, which are described in Part 2 of this book. Macular degeneration is not reversible, but seeing may become easier over time as you adjust to your condition.

Don't try to accept it all in one day or even in one week. This condition will take time to come to grips with, and you may go through a period of sadness and other feelings after you are diagnosed. That is perfectly normal, because you may in a sense be mourning the loss of your vision, and having other personal reactions. (For more information on possible reactions, please see Chapter 9, "Emotional and Psychological Reactions to Age-Related Macular Degeneration.")

It will also take some time to determine what you can still accomplish! Whenever you are in doubt, just read a chapter of this book. Perhaps you will be reminded of a new trick for coping, or you will learn of a new resource to help you. But perhaps most importantly, you will see there is still *hope* for moving on with your life as before, just with some (minor) adjustments.

CHAPTER 2

Look at It This Way

Although being diagnosed with macular degeneration can be a shock, and the news can be overwhelming, there are many ways in which we can continue living the way we want to. There are also a variety of ways to help ourselves through the initial reactions of fear and worry toward a period of adjustment. Talking to family and friends and to doctors we have found to trust and joining support groups too may all help. But of all the resources available to people with macular degeneration, I have found—and you may, too—that a positive outlook, if we can make our way toward it, is more helpful than we can imagine. And, it is very inexpensive!

INITIAL ADJUSTMENTS

I have always tried to find a way to turn a bad situation into a bearable one. In fact, I sometimes like to say that since I can't see any of my wrinkles, I don't have any! A laugh once a day is good for the spirit.

Not everyone feels the way I do at first. But having a positive outlook is worth the effort. This is especially true since the list of day-to-day activities that may become more difficult for you to do on your own will seem to grow as AMD progresses. Just wait until you wish the toothpaste would make it to your toothbrush the first time you try to put it there, or that the labels on your medications could speak and tell you what they are. You may be frustrated by the fact that the placement of control buttons on electronic appliances is not standardized, the way, for example, the placement of numbers on a telephone is.

But there are ways to cope and to "make do." Your medications may not be able to speak up (although there are now recording devices on the market that attach to prescription bottles and let them do just that!), but there are watches and clocks on the market that will tell you the time. Speaking thermometers are also available, and for the truly brave, bathroom scales can tell you your weight (although this may cause you to wish you'd lost your hearing instead!).

One of your biggest challenges may be learning to cope with the loss of doing absolutely everything on your own. In all likelihood, you will need assistance. And often you will have to *ask* for that help. Since people will not necessarily be able to tell that you have AMD by looking at you, many will not be aware you're in need unless you actually tell them.

This happens to me often. Upon looking at me, people have no idea that I have AMD. Since I cannot recognize faces, I often have to say, "Can you please remind me who you are again?" Since being diagnosed, one thing I have had to learn is to speak up when I do not recognize someone. By now, I no longer worry about having to ask someone to reintroduce themselves to me.

In addition, I have learned to ask for help when I need it, which is difficult when you are used to always doing things on your own. Your faith in humanity may even be restored as a result of having AMD. You will see time and time again just how kind and thoughtful people can be, and how much it can mean to them to do something for you.

While having to get help may make you feel as though you've lost all control of your life, in fact, getting the help you need gives you control over the things you want to do and accomplish. And you may find that doing a task or participating in an activity lifts your spirits if you're feeling down.

There will probably be periods when you do feel blue. You may get angry, frustrated, or depressed, or all three at once. You may agonize over the day when AMD may affect your second eye and agonize even more if it finally does. You may hate riding in a car, because once-familiar places are no longer recognizable to you. Even going to the grocery store can be completely frustrating on your own.

Yes, it will be difficult to be in a room full of people and not be able to recognize anyone. You'll probably be frustrated when someone comes up to talk to you and you have no idea who it is. Half the time you may feel dependent; the other half of the time, you may feel isolated.

COMING TO TERMS WITH AMD

Dealing with macular degeneration is not easy; your new condition will probably be hard to accept. But chances are you've faced adversity before. You know that things can be okay. And the bottom line is that for your own sake, you must at some point come to terms with AMD and try to learn how to make the best of it.

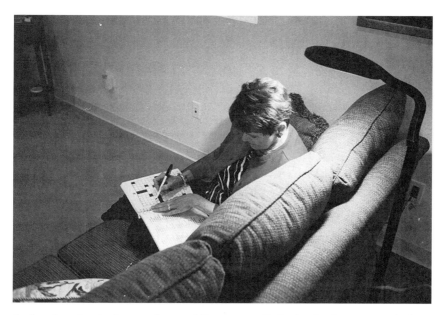

A simple adaptation such as adding more light in the home can help a person with vision loss continue to do favorite activities. (Earl Dotter/ American Foundation for the Blind)

Here are a few tips, based upon my personal experiences:

+ If you find that you are avoiding doing things that are too stressful for you as you react to the news of your diagnosis, it's okay *not* to do them for now. Just don't forget to do them later, when you have adjusted.
+ Go ahead and vent frustration when you feel it.
+ But then consider finding new activities to replace the ones you no longer do. For example, if you can still read, take advantage of online networks and helpful organizations on the Internet. The Internet is an amazing source of support groups and resources for people who have AMD. (See the Resources section at the back of this book for more information.)

✦ Don't become socially isolated! Join a support group. Call a friend or a family member. Arrange to go out and do something that you enjoy. (These first four tips are what my primary physician recommended to me, and I always found them invaluable in helping me to cope with AMD.)

✦ Have appropriate lighting in your home. Adjust the lights so that you can see. Doing this will help with reading and other activities.

✦ Reevaluate what you have on the floor and around your house. Eliminate throw rugs! Be careful about furniture with sharp corners! Your home needs to be comfortable for you, and you can't worry about falling in your house or getting injured.

✦ Wear comfortable shoes! If you're a woman, forget about high heels, which can catch on stairs and curbs, and force you to trip on the grates of sidewalks. (I did, after being diagnosed with AMD.) Shoes need to be comfortable, fit well, and have the proper support for your feet. They also need to be flat and safe, so you don't have to worry about falling. Shoes can still look good, be comfortable, and fit your feet well—even if they are not high heels.

✦ Finally, try to continue doing everything that you possibly can. Yes, you might need to have someone you know help you. But if you enjoy doing something—such as gardening, as an example—and it makes you happy, by all means, try to continue doing it. Your soul will thank you later.

Please remember some of these tips and come back to them often. Although it may take a while at first to accept the arrival of AMD, once you do, you will probably find that there is an abundance of things out there that you can try in order to go on living the kind of life you want, even with AMD. And remember: in the end, trying to maintain hope and a positive outlook can be the most helpful things you can do for yourself.

CHAPTER 3

Keeping Your Body as Healthy as Your Mind

As of this writing, I am 93, and I just started taking a music class. People sometimes ask me what my "secrets" are to living a long and healthy life. What I am about to share is not exactly earth-shattering. But I have learned over the course of my life that you cannot ignore your body, and you need to do some fundamental things in order to live a healthy life. Even if you are feeling distressed or sad over your recent diagnosis of AMD, your body will start feeling the effects immediately if you start following the suggestions in this chapter. And when your body begins to feel better, it's more likely that your emotional health will be too.

LINDY'S GUIDE TO LIVING A HEALTHY LIFE

1. Don't smoke. If you do smoke, try to quit now. If you have never smoked, don't start, no matter what the circumstances. Among the numerous harmful effects of smoking is that it lowers the flow of blood in the eye (which you do not want). Smoking also appears related to the incidence and progression of AMD. (See Chapter 8, "Age-Related Macular Degeneration: Causes and Current Medical Perspectives.")

I write this as a former smoker. I smoked back in the days when it was "cool" to smoke, and people did it without knowing about the long-term side effects on your health and body. One day, years ago, I was in the car with my husband and my first grandson. My husband, who did not smoke, suddenly said to me, "You know we'll have other grandchildren. Do you want to be around to see them? Then you should stop smoking, so that we can enjoy them together."

My husband had never said anything to me before about my smoking. The fact that he voiced his opposition gave me pause. I decided on that day that he was right, and so I decided to stop. It wasn't easy. In fact, it took me a few times before I was finally able to kick the habit. But just as my husband said all of those years ago, I've now been around to watch all of my grandchildren be born and to enjoy them. I credit this partly to the fact that I stopped smoking and have never smoked since.

2. Exercise! It will help you maintain your balance and strength for activities like walking even if you don't see as well as you did. Every bit helps, even if it is a walk around your apartment or lifting a few weights. (The weights can even be heavy cans that you already have in your kitchen cabinet!)

I work out three times a week. I've been doing this for at least 15 years, and I've really seen a difference in how I feel over time. Like everyone else, as I've gotten older, I've noticed more aches and pains in my body. It doesn't matter the time of day; sometimes I have a mysterious ache or pain for no reason at all!

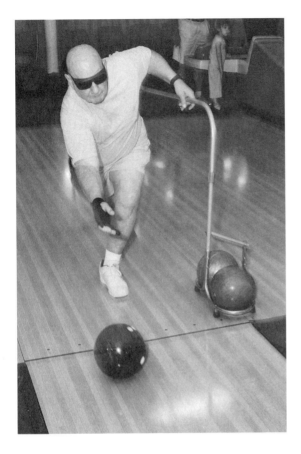

Exercising, however you can do it, is important for your health and balance. Losing one's vision does not mean one has to stop being active. (Earl Dotter/American Foundation for the Blind)

However, I know that I'm stronger now and my body is more resistant to these aches and pains because I exercise. In fact, I'm better about exercising now than I ever was before. Sometimes my exercise consists of swimming, and other times just doing leg bending and other stretching exercises. Other times, I just walk around my apartment or around the block with a friend holding my arm. Sometimes I lift weights.

Whatever you do will help you. The point is not to sit around all day being inactive. It doesn't have to cost anything to exercise; you don't have to join a gym or pay an expensive trainer. And you can work out with a friend, which can provide more motivation than doing it on your own.

Just because you may be losing your vision doesn't mean you can't still exercise like a sighted person. For instance, I know a gentleman who is completely blind. He runs miles through the park a few times a week. How does he do it, you ask? He has two running buddies! He goes with one of his two running buddies often. The friend holds his arm and guides him, so he doesn't trip on a curb. He has been doing this for years, loves it, and people tell me he is extremely trim and fit.

Exercise is also a good stress reliever. Whenever I have had a stressful day, I exercise. I am constantly amazed by how much better I feel after I exercise, and whatever it was that was bothering me doesn't seem to be as upsetting.

So, friends, get moving! No matter what age you are, it's never too late to begin exercising. Your body and health will be greatly rewarded.

3. Vitamins! Studies have shown that vitamins can work if you already have *at least* moderately severe macular degeneration. One study in particular is especially interesting. The Age-Related Eye Disease Study (AREDS), sponsored by the National Eye Institute (see the website at www.nei.nih.gov/amd for a description of the study), showed that a daily supplement of 500 milligrams (mg) of vitamin C, 400 international units (IU) of vitamin E, 15 mg of beta carotene, 80 mg of zinc (as zinc oxide), and 2 mg of copper (as cupric oxide) reduced the risk of AMD progressing from moderate or severe vision loss by up to 25 percent.[1]

The initial AREDS did not study lutein, or other antioxidants, so we don't know how they may affect eye disease. Future clinical trials may eventually provide answers about these and other antioxidants. (The NEI has launched the Age-Related Eye Disease Study 2 [AREDS2]; see www.areds2.org.[2] The new study reduced the originally recommended amount of zinc to 40 mg. For more information, see Chapter 8.) Note that in the initial AREDS study, it was found that people with mild or early stages of AMD did *not* benefit from taking these supplements.

In addition, there are many health benefits to taking fish oil, which is found in high concentrations in fish like salmon, herring, and sardines. These types of fish contain good levels of omega-3 fatty acids. Personally, I'm not a big fan of sardines, so I take fish oil supplements. They are usually easy to find, in the same store aisle as multivitamins. In any event, you should also talk to your doctor first before taking fish oil supplements if you're at risk for AMD.

A recent study from Harvard, called the Harvard Women's Health Study, which was published in the *Archives of Ophthalmology,* reported that "women whose diets were rich in omega-3 fatty acids found in fish were at significantly lower risk of developing age-related macular degeneration."[3] The study followed thousands of women in midlife over an average of 10 years. The analysis found that women who reported "eating one or more servings of fish per week were 42 percent less likely to develop AMD than those who ate less than a serving each month. (Researchers adjusted the data to control for other factors linked to the disease, including smoking.) Eating canned tuna and dark-meat fish like mackerel, salmon, sardines, bluefish and swordfish appeared to have the most benefit."

4. Eat brightly colored fruits and vegetables every day. I keep hearing about how important it is to eat several servings of fruit and vegetables every day. For example, the American Heart Association recommends eating eight or more fruit and vegetable servings every day and has said that an average adult consuming 2,000 calories daily should aim to eat 4.5 cups of fruits and vegetables daily.

The more brightly colored the fruits and vegetables are, the better they apparently are for you! They are particularly good for the eyes and help maintain your overall eye health. Here's an example. Spinach and kale are a much brighter and darker green than white-to-light-green iceberg lettuce, and they contain much higher levels of antioxidants and vitamins. You might therefore use my easy-to-remember rule: The brighter it is, the healthier it is for you. (I'm talking only about naturally colored fruits and vegetables—nothing artificially colored or enhanced.) Other "gold star" vegetables include tomatoes, broccoli, red peppers, carrots, and romaine lettuce.

Although it may be difficult at first, try to make a concerted effort to eat more brightly colored vegetables, like spinach, and ease off on the iceberg lettuce, which contains much more water and substantially fewer vitamins. You can eat these vegetables either fresh or frozen to add variety to your meals. To help make your choices more interesting, you can make it a red/green/purple day (apple, dark green lettuce leaf, purple grapes) or see if you can consume a rainbow of fruits and vegetables during the week.

And please try to stay away from drowning your vegetables in butter, cheese, or thick and rich salad dressing. Also try to avoid salad toppings that add only fat and calories with no nutritional value (like bacon bits and high-fat croutons). Otherwise, you might end up "undoing" some of the wonderful things that vegetables do for us! In addition, try to use healthier cooking methods. Steaming, grilling, sautéing, roasting, baking, and microwaving vegetables are ideal preparation methods. Try not to use butter or to fry your food.

Finally, there are some fruits that are particularly high in antioxidants. They include the berry family: strawberries, blueberries, raspberries, and blackberries. Try to include them in your diet whenever possible each day. Berries are easy to sneak into your meals. For instance, you can top your morning cereal or yogurt snack with fresh berries. You can also dress up any spinach salad with sliced strawberries, cranberries, broccoli, slivered almonds, and a splash of balsamic vinegar. For an easy, elegant dessert, blend fresh or frozen berries with a spoonful of honey and some frozen yogurt. Freeze for 20 minutes, then spoon into serving cups and decorate with a sprig of mint.

I know one person who, when she can't sleep at night, actually counts how many servings a day she has of fruits and vegetables. She aims for 8 to 10 servings of vegetables and fruit daily. While that might be a little unrealistic for a lot of people, start slowly by sneaking fruits and vegetables into your meals and snacks. Pretty soon, you may not think twice about having baby carrots as a snack, instead of potato chips, and having strawberries in your yogurt instead of splurging your calories on a candy bar.

5. *See your eye doctor regularly.* The risk of getting macular degeneration increases with age. If you haven't been to your eye doctor for a few years, it's possible to have macular degeneration without even knowing it. Unfortunately, macular degeneration progresses silently, and our eyes are designed to compensate for each other when one cannot see as well as the other. As a result, vision can sometimes be lost from macular degeneration without an individual realizing it. An ophthalmologist (an eye doctor) can detect the early signs of macular degeneration before you lose any vision. Accordingly, you should see your eye doctor at least once a year. It's all part of keeping your eyes (and body) as healthy as your mind.

NOTES

1. Age-Related Eye Disease Study Research Group, "A Randomized, Placebo-Controlled, Clinical Trial of High-Dose Supplementation with Vitamins C and E, Beta Carotene, and Zinc for Age-Related Macular Degeneration and Vision Loss," AREDS Report no. 8, *Archives of Ophthalmology* 119 (October 2001): 1417–36.

2. Age-Related Eye Disease Study Research Group, "A Randomized, Placebo-Controlled, Clinical Trial of High-Dose Supplementation with Vitamins C and E and Beta Carotene for Age-Related Cataract and Vision Loss," AREDS Report no. 9, *Archives of Ophthalmology* 119 (October 2001): 1439–52.

3. William G. Christen, Debra A. Schaumberg, Robert J. Glynn, and Julie E. Buring, "Dietary Omega-3 Fatty Acid and Fish Intake and Incident Age-Related Macular Degeneration in Women," *Archives of Ophthalmology.* Published online March 14, 2011, http://archopht.ama-assn.org. Cited in Roni Caryn Rabin, "Diet: Eating Fish Found to Ward Off Eye Disease," *New York Times*, March 22, 2011, D6.

CHAPTER 4

Life with Less Vision, and How to Move Forward

In order to function without full vision, you may need to be creative. So, now is the time to learn some new tricks. I adjusted to life with less vision and learned a lot through trial and error, and now I am sharing some of what I learned with you! The following are my five top tips from my reservoir bank.

TIP NO. 1: ORGANIZE YOUR LIFE NOW

After you are diagnosed with AMD, you may want to make a list of items you will need to do while you still can. For example, get a statement of your eye condition from your doctor. Make copies of it so that if you ever need to verify that you have AMD, you can provide the statement as proof. This statement can help you on many levels. For example, in many states, you can get telephone directory assistance for free or at a reduced rate if you are blind or visually impaired. You will need proof for your telephone company or service provider, so this statement from your doctor may be essential later on.

Also, get your home organized so you know where things are. Finding a specific place for everything you need

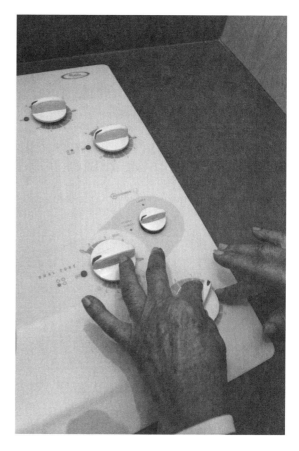

Marking the settings of appliances with stickers or color-coded raised dots that you can feel will help with everyday tasks around the house. (Earl Dotter/American Foundation for the Blind)

and putting things back when you are finished using them will cure more headaches than aspirin!

You can also symbol- and color-code your appliances and can use larger-sized stickers that contain different colors or symbols. For instance, you can put a green sticker near the 350-degree marker on the stove, and a red sticker by the off button. These stickers can help you to know where items are in your kitchen when you look at the colors of or the symbols on the stickers.

Stickers like these will be easier to see than the small type found on electronic control panels. Stickers in different colors, with various symbols and textures, are available at drug stores, office supply shops, and low vision device centers, such as the store at The Chicago Lighthouse (and through its website at www.chicagolighthouse.org; also see the Resources section). Craft supply stores also sell various stickers (even rhinestone stickers!) of all shapes and sizes that you can use. (I put a pink rhinestone sticker on my phone on the number "zero," so I can easily feel where it is.)

Finally, address the issue of who's going to help you deal with the details of your life. You're going to have to get through your mail, for example, and pay all your bills. How will you deposit money in the bank, and what will you do about groceries when and if you reach the point where you cannot shop on your own?

Once you figure out how you will get these things accomplished, you may feel more comfortable accepting your new circumstances. You may need to turn to your family, dear friends, and trusted colleagues to help you figure this all out. You can also check out the Resources section of this book for different agencies that perhaps can help you as well. In fact, see the next tip below.

TIP NO. 2: OBTAIN ASSISTANCE FROM AN AGENCY THAT HELPS PEOPLE WHO ARE VISUALLY IMPAIRED

As you may know, there are not-for-profit organizations all over the country that specifically help people with visual impairments. A list of some of the national organizations and agencies that could potentially assist you is in the Resources section in the back of this book. There are many more that are not listed, and you might want to check the *AFB Directory of Services* mentioned in that section, or call the American Foundation for the Blind or other organizations listed and ask them about a local agency in your area.

One agency in particular, The Chicago Lighthouse, has assisted me over the years, and it has given me tremendous hope and help. The Chicago Lighthouse has, at last count, 28 programs and services to help people who are blind or visually impaired. No one is turned away due to their inability to pay. If The Chicago Lighthouse, or one of its sister agencies around the country, is not located near you, you might still call it, and perhaps a staff member can refer you to an agency near where you live that can help you.

One program that a lot of my friends who have AMD truly enjoy is a radio reading service, which is a reading service for blind and visually impaired listeners. This is a service offered by charitable organizations, universities, community groups, and public radio stations, in which a narrator reads books, newspapers, and magazines aloud for the benefit of people who are blind or visually impaired or who have other disabilities. It is most often broadcast over the radio, usually on otherwise unused frequencies, and a special radio receiver permanently tuned to a given station in the area is used to pick up the closed-circuit broadcast. Some reading services use alternative methods for reaching their audiences, including broadcasting over streaming or archived Internet radio, cable TV, or telephone dial-in systems.

The International Association of Audio Information Services (IAAIS) is the worldwide organization of over 100 independent audio information services that provide printed material in audio form through closed-circuit radio broadcasts, dial-in telephone newspaper systems, personal recording, and Internet broadcasting and program archives.

In almost all cases, these services are provided free of charge. You can call the IAAIS National Office (see Resources) or access them on the Internet. Online, there is a comprehensive list of all IAAIS member radio information services in Canada and the United States, with links to their individual websites. You can find this list at www.iaais .org/findservices.html.

The Chicago Lighthouse has its own free radio service. It is called Chicagoland Radio Information Services, and is known as CRIS. It provides daily readings of newspapers and periodicals, including news stories, sales circulars, and classified listings for listeners who have a wide range of disabilities. Mainly through the use of volunteers, CRIS broadcasts verbatim readings of the *Chicago Tribune, Chicago Sun-Times,* and many more newspapers and magazines. It also broadcasts audio-described movies, in which descriptions of what is happening on screen are provided, and produces special interest programming dedicated to serving the interests of its visually impaired and disabled community. Tens of thousands of listeners tune in from special receivers placed in private residences, schools, libraries, hospitals, nursing homes, retirement centers, hospices, and community centers.

CRIS broadcasts to the world via live audio streaming online. By clicking on the "CRIS" icon on The Chicago Lighthouse's website, listeners have access to the same printed information available to people without vision loss. Special interest programs are also available for downloads and podcasts. If you have access to the Internet, you also have access to CRIS's free service through the link for CRIS at www.chicagolighthouse.org. You can also obtain a schedule of the programming online.

You may also find it helpful to know about The Lighthouse's Tools for Living store in Chicago. This amazing store has everything to help you be independent in your own home, from independent living aids to kitchen devices, portable reading devices, and even tactile toys for your grandchildren. The store was designed for people with low vision, and there are special nonglare lighting and color-contrasting displays that allow you to see items easily. In addition, the people who work in the store are trained to guide and help each person and family members as they choose the items that are most appropriate for their needs. Even if you do not live in Chicago, you can still visit the store by going online at www.chicagolighthouse.org/store. In addition, many of the organizations found in the *AFB Directory of Services* and in this book's Resources section have stores to help you as well, and there are a number of catalogs and companies online that sell products that help people with low vision live independently.

TIP NO. 3: KNOW THAT *YOU CAN STILL READ!*

Today, there are many ways to read and access print materials, such as electronic books, audio books, and large-print materials. For instance, for those using a computer, an organization called Bookshare (whose website is www .bookshare.org) has a program especially for persons who are blind or visually impaired. Once registered for a nominal fee, a person can download up to 100 books per month. These books can be read on a computer with screen enlargement software or a screen reader software program (which Bookshare provides for free) or can be downloaded into a portable device that stores the books and electronically converts them into synthetic speech.

There are all sorts of large-print books available, including cookbooks. Your local library has them, and they are also available at bookstores and online. There are also large-print magazines available, like *Reader's Digest.* Many of the people I know who read them say they are extremely helpful. Now devices such as e-book readers and tablet computers can accept books and magazines that are instantly downloaded onto the device. The user can choose any size print, including giant print for all books and magazines. Many devices also offer the option to read the material aloud. In addition, smartphones (mobile phones that can perform many functions) can use applications that also allow downloading of books directly onto the phone with large-type and audio options.

Loved by many is the *Matilda Ziegler Magazine.* It is a longtime publication that was formerly available via large print and braille and now is available only online, at www .matildaziegler.com. It describes itself as "a well-rounded blend of general interest news and blindness-related information specifically made for the blind and visually impaired." It also presents events going on around the country, as well as articles on the latest in adaptive technology. If you would like to subscribe to *Matilda Ziegler's* weekly e-mail edition, a compilation of each week's postings to the site, you can do so at the website.

Another reading option is to use audio books (which used to be called "books on tape") to help keep your mind active and to keep literature in your life. You can find audio books at local libraries, which will lend them to you free of charge. They are also readily available at bookstores or can be ordered through catalogs. You will also find that a wide range of magazines are recorded for people who are blind or visually impaired.

An important reading program is also offered by the U.S. Library of Congress, which, for free, sends audio books and magazines to registered users. You can even specify what types of books you want sent to you (such as new fiction, mysteries, or romance). Inquire at your local library for an application for the National Library Service (NLS) Talking Book Program. They should have one, or if not, they can help direct you to one. (You can also see the Resources section for more information. You can get a list of local libraries from the NLS or from AFB's *Directory of Services*.) A letter from your eye doctor is needed to certify that your vision loss keeps you from reading print materials. Once approved, you will get the machine you need to use for free. Persons who use a computer can also access the National Library Service books online through its website at www.loc.gov/nls. I know many people who love the Library of Congress Talking Books, including me!

One new "toy" I recently found at my public library is a device that contains one preloaded, digital, portable Talking Book. It is lightweight, weighing only two ounces, and is about half the size of a deck of cards, but it will hold an entire book, up to 60 hours of playtime. It allows the listener to control the speed of the narrator's voice, and it automatically bookmarks the last place you left off after powering down. All you need is a pair of headphones that you plug into the audio book, then you hit "play" and listen to the story! What a great idea: just plug in your own earphones, and you are ready to go! Given how quickly changes are taking place in technology today, these and many other devices probably soon will be available for all of us to use at no or minimal cost.

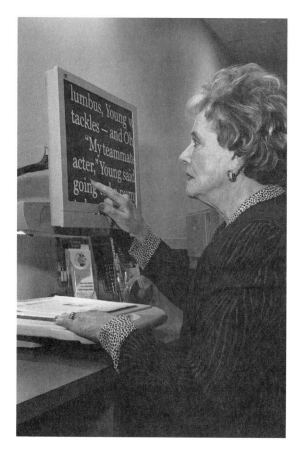

There are a variety of ways to continue reading, including using a closed-circuit television system (CCTV) or video magnifier, like this one, that enlarges text and can change its color to make it easier to view. (Earl Dotter/American Foundation for the Blind)

Finally, many people use reading machines, such as closed-circuit televisions, or CCTVs, which are also called video magnifiers. These devices illuminate and magnify images and words on a screen to help you see them. You may never read *Anna Karenina* on this kind of machine, but it is relatively good for reading the mail. Reading machines are, however, one of the more expensive low vision devices on the market, although prices have declined in recent years. Today, a variety of machines is available, in all sizes and for all budgets. I like using my CCTV because it allows me to be independent. There are even portable video magnifiers available now, which you can take with you and use to read the menus in restaurants or labels in grocery stores. (For more on CCTVs and other forms of adaptive technology, please see Chapter 11 in this book).

TIP NO. 4: MAKE SURE YOU COMMUNICATE WITH OTHERS

For persons experiencing vision loss, it is important to keep in touch with family and friends and avoid a feeling of isolation. The telephone is an excellent tool, and so is a computer. Today, we all use computers for so much more than writing notes or paying bills. Computers and other forms of technology have transformed the way we live and work. If you use a computer, in most cases, you can make the images on the screen as large and plain as you like, and your fingers may already know the keyboard, but large-print keys or stick-on keytops are now available.

If enlarging the images on the screen is not helpful to you, you can try using screen-reading software, which announces or "reads" the information on the screen and makes it available using synthesized speech and/or refreshable braille. Refreshable braille is a method of converting text on the computer screen into braille, using an electronic device consisting of plastic pins that pop up to form braille characters. Screen-reading software is not hard to install, and when you use it, you perform all functions on the computer exclusively using the keyboard. You can change the voice, speech rate, and even the language in which the machine speaks to you. With screen-reading software, you can do everything on the computer that a sighted person can do, even if you cannot see the screen! (For more about adaptive technology, please see Chapter 11).

Communicating on the telephone is virtually unaffected by AMD. You may have to learn to dial or touch your phone's keypad without looking, but phones with large numbers, quick-dial capability, and program options are readily available. Many cell phones now have a voice-dialing capability, and many models have a touch screen and built-in screen magnifier and text-to-speech capabilities. And, as mentioned earlier, directory assistance on your home phone may offer free special services for people who are visually impaired; calling your phone company to inquire may be helpful.

And after you've talked to all your friends and family members, get in touch with other people who have macular degeneration. You may not be longing for someone to relate to, but often in life it is the people who have experienced what we are going through who seem to be the most helpful sources of information, advice, and support. Ask your doctor about other groups or individuals you may find valuable to contact. There may even be a person who would benefit from talking to you. This is one way you can still do something for someone else—and it may also do something for you.

I think it is extremely important to have a cell or mobile phone, especially if you are going out alone. A cell phone is good for meeting someone, and it can give you a sense of security. Several manufacturers are beginning to offer cell phones with large keys and displays for seniors. The one that I have, the Jitterbug, like any other phone, may not be completely problem-free, but friendly operators place calls for you. The Jitterbug has large, tactile dials and also includes a service where you can ask an operator for any type of help. Again, a letter from your eye doctor may help lessen the cost of this type of service when you first apply.

Watching television is another way of staying connected to the world. The television may be difficult to watch, but there are solutions. For example, there are TV glasses, available through many low vision clinics or low vision optometrists, that work like low-powered binoculars. They have a focus ring on the side of each temple, which is adjustable for each eye.

Another possibility may be to rearrange the furniture to sit in close proximity to the TV screen. The television is best viewed at eye level when you have AMD. In addition, a huge screen is not needed if you are sitting very close to the television.

The radio can be useful as well. You may be surprised at the variety of programming on the air throughout the day. There is also satellite radio, which offers hundreds of channels in every sort of music and talk radio genre conceivable. It is available by subscription only but is affordable. You can also get a satellite receiver that has user-friendly buttons and is also available in the car. Shortwave radio can also be very entertaining. You can even get the BBC and Vatican City Radio, among other stations.

But don't become a couch potato. And if you've always been one, try changing that. Activities will help give you confidence, help you stay connected to others, and may keep you from worrying about your eyes and any possible vision loss.

To attend cultural events, which is generally not out of the question, try using special telescopic lenses available for people who are visually impaired. They're not perfect, but they're fairly unobtrusive and they work pretty well at concerts and lectures. There are several types, some called sport scopes, that you wear like tiny binocular glasses. Other more sophisticated telescopes are called bioptic telescopes. They work like regular prescription eyeglasses but have a tiny telescope mounted near the top of a single lens used with your better-seeing eye. They are available only by prescription through low vision optometrists or a low vision center. (See Chapter 10, "The Low Vision Eye Exam," for more information.)

To get exercise, try swimming. Many people close their eyes when they swim anyway, and you're probably in a relatively safe environment when you're in the pool. Besides, swimming is a great workout, and it is a good outlet for making new friends.

In addition, as already mentioned, many people benefit from attending a support group. You can make new friends and may find you can feel comfortable discussing your trials and tribulations because you know others can relate. You can also share insights and successes, which could be invaluable to others in the group. I've joined a few groups throughout the years, and they helped me tremendously. Support groups have been lifesavers for many people dealing with a wide range of issues. They are certainly worth exploring for people with macular degeneration. The Association for Macular Diseases and Macular Degeneration International are examples of organizations that offer support groups for individuals and their families with macular degeneration. (See the Resources section at the back of this book for information about these organizations.)

You may be able to find others by searching online, by checking with any agency that has been providing you services, or by consulting the resource list at the back of this book. Your doctor may also be able to help you locate resources that are right for you.

TIP NO. 5: CONSIDER USING A WHITE CANE!

Canes are often used by visually impaired people who have received special training with them from an orientation and mobility (O&M) instructor. O&M instruction is designed to help individuals with low vision travel safely and independently and is often part of low vision services (see Chapter 10). Whether you have formal O&M training or not, you may want to consider using a long white cane when you go out in public. While you may have to adjust to the idea that you're carrying a cane, this is one way to alert people to the fact that you can't see very well, if they know what a white cane signifies. The cane can even be empowering, because it often commands respect on the

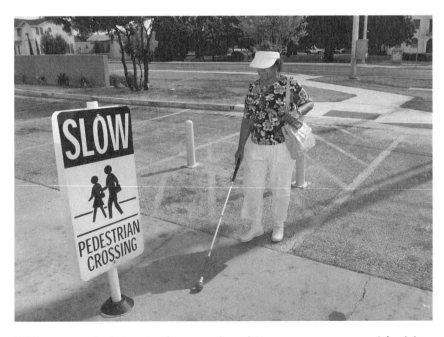

With proper training in the use of a white cane, a person with vision loss can learn to travel safely and independently. (Earl Dotter/American Foundation for the Blind)

street. You may even feel a sense of security when you carry it. The cane also helps you with balance. In addition, it can help you feel how deep something is as you are walking, like the depth of a curb. Finally, the cane also reminds people who know you that you have a visual impairment, which means you don't have to announce it all the time. But keep track of the cane. It's easy to leave behind.

I thought I would close this chapter with a few inspirational quotes from Helen Keller, a great lady who lived with vision and hearing loss in an inspiring way. She gave us so many inspiring lines, it was difficult to pick just a few:

"The best and most beautiful things in the world cannot be seen or even touched. They must be felt with the heart."

"Alone we can do so little; together we can do so much."

"Optimism is the faith that leads to achievement. Nothing can be done without hope and confidence."

CHAPTER 5

Consider the Family

The family and friends of a person with AMD play an incredibly significant role. Doctors will often turn to family members to ask who's going to help you get along. If your lines of communication have broken down, now is the time to rebuild them.

You can help this process by trying to be open and honest with people, including yourself, although it may be difficult at first. You may want to deny the fact that you have AMD. But since you're seeing the eye doctor regularly and you have a diagnosis of the disease, try to acknowledge that you have AMD. Doing this will help you begin your new life and can help you move forward.

HOW COMMUNICATION CAN BE KEY

Living with AMD can be made easier if you communicate with your friends and family about the disease. Tell them what's going on. Try to describe the physical effects you are experiencing, and point out for them just what you can and can't see at each stage. Explain that it's weird: sometimes you can see a thread on the carpet, while most times you can't see the person you're talking to. Suggest that they hold their hands in front of their eyes. As they stare straight ahead, ask them what they see in their peripheral vision. This might give them an idea of what you can see.

Discussing your condition can be hard, because most people, including you, probably don't have a frame of reference for impaired vision. Actually being able to convey what you see through words may prove tricky. But give it a shot. And try to express how you feel about it all. Explore the range of emotions you've experienced, and listen to those of others. And, finally, although it may be difficult, try to talk about the needs you have and where you feel dependent. The more you share with those around you, the better they can understand your condition, and the easier it may be for everyone!

Everyone will need to adjust. You will probably have to come to terms with depending on others, rather than having them depend on you. You will probably also need to find the courage to ask people to identify themselves when they approach you. Finally, though it may take some time, you will probably need to learn to accept help from others.

If you do not have family and friends as a resource, there are still alternatives and support available. You can talk to your doctors, seek out counseling, join a support group, and look for help from not-for-profit organizations that assist people who are blind or visually impaired, just to name a few options. (Please see the Resources section for more options.)

ADJUSTMENT IS AN ONGOING PROCESS

Everybody may end up feeling guilty at some point. You may feel guilty for taking out your frustrations on people or for imposing on their time. They may feel guilty, because they think they don't do enough for you.

You may also feel an internal struggle about wanting to ask for help yet still wanting to do things on your own. You may also not want to be a "burden" to anyone. This is where it helps to have some adaptive technology, like a CCTV or video magnifier in your house, so that you can still read your friends' telephone numbers independently. Or get a Jitterbug phone, so if you want to call a friend and can't read the phone number, the operator on the other end will put the call through for you.

Of course, it's much faster to have someone read the numbers to me or dial the phone. But I feel I need to do some things on my own. So, I use my CCTV to look up my friends' phone numbers, and I use my regular house phone to dial the numbers, since I know where the numbers are on the phone. In addition, someone kindly made me my own list of telephone numbers, Lindy's List. It is in a large font (14 point), in bold, and I look at it under my CCTV to read my most important numbers. It is in a three-ring binder, so I can replace the list as it needs to be updated.

It is important to maintain some sense of independence if possible, and being able to do some things on your own helps with that important goal. On the other hand, you also need to understand the limits of what you can do. Accordingly, I often have a friend grocery-shop with me during the week, since I can no longer do that by myself.

This will all be part of learning to cope with AMD. Macular degeneration certainly has its negative side, but one good thing about it is that it can sometimes encourage people to become more introspective and sympathetic. Think about the impact vision loss is having on you. Try to understand that your family and friends have to come to terms with your condition, too. Try to be realistic about your expectations, and be gentle with yourself and others.

It is almost inevitable that everyone involved with AMD will be changed in some way. When you or your loved ones behave atypically, try to analyze why. And remember, there are no quick answers. You will need patience, and to give everyone (including yourself!) some time to absorb the AMD diagnosis and to understand how it will affect your life.

CHAPTER 6

A Note to Loved Ones

In times of trouble, it is family and friends who make a difference in how well a person gets along. Here are some relatively easy ways for friends and family to help:

✦ Offering to do the basics is a nice gesture. Bringing over dinner, running errands, and offering to do grocery shopping are great ways to help people with AMD.

✦ So is offering an arm to hold while crossing the street. For instance, I try not to go anywhere outside of my house without having my white cane and an arm to guide me. I just can't take the risk of falling or becoming lost.

✦ If you see someone walking alone with a white cane, please offer to help the person. He or she may not need assistance and may say no, thank you. But the simple gesture of helping someone who is blind or visually impaired and who does need some support in this way can mean a great deal to a person who might otherwise struggle to get across the street on his or her own.

In addition, such simple acts as describing something in detail so that the person can imagine it can mean a lot. And so can encouraging him or her to touch objects, including the faces of grandchildren, to get a better sense of them. I do that often with my grandchildren. A nice gift for a person with AMD might be something that smells good, like flowers or a new bath soap. And remember to call your loved one often!

Other thoughtful things to do for someone with AMD include these:

♦ Saying your name when you approach someone with AMD, so he or she knows who you are. (Very important! If you can't see someone's face, you need another way of identifying that person. People with AMD appreciate this small gesture, and it only takes a moment to do.)

♦ Making recordings of favorite songs and familiar voices.

♦ Setting the microwave so that all someone has to do is retrieve a prepared meal from the refrigerator and hit the start button (and perhaps marking where the start button is with a sticker that the person can feel). This way he or she can eat when it's convenient.

♦ Helping the person keep busy in meaningful ways. For example, invitations to excursions are probably welcome. But the kind of activity should be given consideration; for instance, a movie may not be as good an idea as a concert. Plan the outing with the individual in mind! For someone who loves reading, a bookstore may be fine if there is an audio section. Just call ahead to make sure!

♦ Printing in large letters rather than using cursive handwriting when writing something to be read by a person with AMD. Also, use a bold, felt-tipped marker of some kind, such as a 20/20 pen.

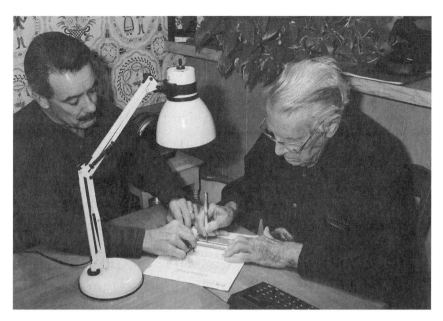

Helping with household chores, such as paying the bills, is one way for friends and family members to assist a person with AMD. (Earl Dotter/American Foundation for the Blind)

In general and if possible, friends and family should try to note their loved one's subtle behavior, such as a particular attitude and silent struggles. Sometimes it's the things left unsaid that say the most.

When it comes to the children in a family, consider macular degeneration a learning experience, as it is for everyone. It's good to explain the situation to them and help them understand how they can contribute. A favorite for young readers, for example, is to be allowed to read menus (don't forget the prices) or road signs for the person with AMD. Children also like to guide their loved one when walking—but they should be reminded to lead and not pull the person. Also, ask the person first whether he or she would like to take your arm or have an arm held. If it is the latter, then asking which arm is preferred is especially considerate.

For instance, I like to hold onto people. I always take someone's arm; I feel more secure that way. I also appreciate it when people ask me at the outset which of their arms would work better for me to hold onto.

AMD is a good opportunity for children to learn compassion and acceptance. It's a chance for them to see firsthand that adversity can be managed and that you can still live a happy and meaningful life. Most important, family and friends can help their loved one to have a good attitude. Laughter still is the best medicine, and love from beloved friends and family still can help heal the pain.

In the end, a diagnosis of macular degeneration may be daunting, but it is not a death sentence. Still listen closely for the sound of music! What you can still hear will amaze you (even if you are in your 90s!)

Afterword

A Point of View

Lindy Bergman with Jennifer E. Miller

When Lindy Bergman was first diagnosed with AMD, the specialist told Lindy, "But you will be able to manage."

Lindy never forgot these words. And for three years, she did manage quite well. But then AMD affected her other eye. Then she began to have to change her life.

"I'm no authority," Lindy says. "I can only share my own experiences. But maybe I can make suggestions that will help others get along better."

It's easy for her, you may say, because Lindy has been fortunate in her life and is an optimist by nature. But the loss of her vision is, in fact, something that hit Lindy very close to home.

For many years, she and her husband, Ed, invested a lot of time in learning about art. Initially excited by an art course they took, Lindy and Ed embraced contemporary artworks. They surrounded themselves with art they enjoyed collecting together, and it was a passion they shared with great enthusiasm.

As a result, Lindy's adjustment to macular degeneration was not easy. Perhaps reconciling vision loss for someone who is so visually oriented can be particularly difficult.

But despite that, she persevered. And in her case, she believes that coping with AMD made her stronger. Although she may not be able to see her artwork clearly today, Lindy still enjoys her art, because she remembers it. And even though Lindy may have forgotten exact pictures, she can remember a lot about them, how she obtained them, and stories about the artists she met. Just thinking about some of the pieces makes her smile today.

"It's been a challenge for me," Lindy says. "But I've personally found that my best defense is humor, and I've always relied on hope. These have served me well. My life goes on. I can still enjoy it, and I'm grateful, because I have had a lot of help. I have been especially thankful for my supportive family and friends over the years. And if I laugh a little each day, I find it keeps me going a long way."

PART 2

Professional Perspectives

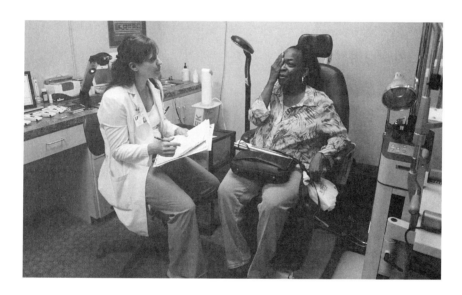

Prologue

Janet P. Szlyk

It has been a joy getting to know Lindy Bergman outside of The Chicago Lighthouse, where she has been a client and friend of the agency for a number of years. I especially enjoy sharing meals and personal stories at our favorite French restaurant on Taylor Street. Over salmon and *pomme frites,* we have talked about family, work, history, travel, and art. I always end our delightful times together thinking how positive and genuinely happy she is, and also wondering how a woman who had dedicated such a significant part of her life to collecting works of visual art could adapt so well to the loss of the ability to see them. As we've become friends, I realize that what makes Lindy so interesting is her intelligence and keen interest in everyone and everything. With Lindy, it's not about her; she is much more interested in hearing what is happening with you. After almost three years, I now feel that I have a better understanding of the force of optimism that is Lindy Bergman, and some of the secrets to her resilient spirit. She is also a shining example of a person whose visual sensory system might have faltered, but who through experience has archived wonderful memories in her brain to compensate!

The disorder that has affected her vision is age-related macular degeneration (AMD), which is a leading cause of blindness in people over the age of 65 years.[1] The disease causes a deterioration of the central, or macular, region of the retina and results in a loss of the ability to resolve fine detail. Tasks such as reading or recognizing faces become difficult. The estimates of those impacted are startling, with one in three persons over 75 years affected by the disease.[2] More are being affected as the 79 million baby boomers reach or near retirement age.

There are significant breakthroughs being made in the treatment of the disease, including the highly effective agent Lucentis, the injectable drug ranibizumab, which appears to inhibit further growth of new blood vessels that rob vision in the "wet" form of AMD. Gene therapies for this neovascular type of AMD are being developed and tested. Miniature telescopic lens implants show improved vision and promise for some older patients affected by the "dry" type of AMD that is characterized by decay of the central macular region without the growth of new vessels. Special vitamin formulas have been demonstrated in controlled studies to delay the progression of the "dry" type of AMD in some patients. There are also significant advances being made in the functional rehabilitation of patients who are experiencing macular degeneration.

As a scientist in the field of vision rehabilitation, my research interests have been focused on the development of new methods to help patients optimize their remaining vision. Anecdotally, I noticed that patients were not able to take advantage of new behavioral therapies or to learn to use optical enhancement devices if they were depressed or were having difficulty adjusting to their progressive vision loss. It was a fairly frequent occurrence to encounter

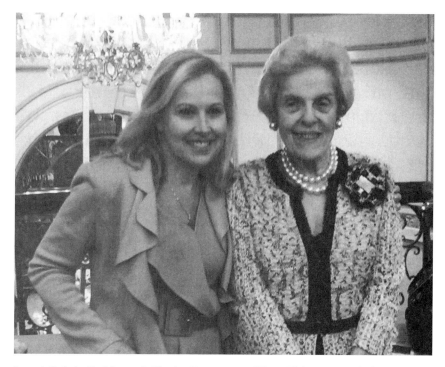

Janet Szlyk (left) and Lindy Bergman (The Chicago Lighthouse for People Who Are Blind or Visually Impaired)

patients who had entered a research study in my laboratory who stated that they were having problems adjusting to the changes in their vision and were experiencing depressive symptoms. They would then be referred to general mental health specialists.

I often thought it would be much better for patients if their psychological rehabilitation could be done in conjunction with their vision rehabilitation in the same environment. It was a hope of mine to make this a reality, but there was a major obstacle in the dearth of mental health professionals whose practices focused on patients with visual impairments. It is important to note that there were few, if any, specialists in the major metropolitan area of Chicago, home to over six million people, with a unique expertise or specialty in treating the depression that occurs with the loss of one's vision.

In reviewing the literature, one can find studies showing that nearly one-third of patients with AMD had feelings of depression. These findings, and observation of our own patients, prompted our laboratory to directly investigate the impact of depression on rehabilitation outcomes. We recently documented the perhaps not surprising finding that patients who were experiencing depressive symptoms had significantly poorer outcomes in a reading rehabilitation program.[3] This translated into worse reading speed scores following training. The obvious implication to us is that it does not make sense to have a rehabilitation program without a psychological component.

Despite this evidence that many patients with AMD suffer depression and emotional trauma, a psychological consultation is not standard practice in rehabilitation programs. Furthermore, patients are not often being referred to a mental health professional when given their life-changing diagnosis. In fact, in a recent article in a leading journal in the field, fewer than 5 percent of low vision rehabilitation services in the United States have programs that include a professional trained to deal with the emotional sequelae associated with AMD.[4] However, the same article reports that nearly half the clients (44.9 percent) of rehabilitation services were described as having problems with emotional or psychological adjustment, and an average of 67.1 percent of clients had a diagnosis of AMD.

THE CHICAGO LIGHTHOUSE MODEL

The Chicago Lighthouse has the distinction of being one of the first eye care centers in the United States that focused on patients with low vision. Our clinic was dedicated by Helen Keller in 1956. The founding father of our clinic, Dr.

Alfred Rosenbloom, hosted Ms. Keller at the ceremony. Dr. Rosenbloom still practices and holds the prestigious Krumrey Chair in Low Vision. Interestingly, Dr. Elisabeth Kübler-Ross, the psychiatrist famous for describing the stages of adaptation and grief associated with death and dying—denial, anger, bargaining, depression, and acceptance[5]—was inspired by her observations of patients losing their vision at The Chicago Lighthouse. Dr. Kübler-Ross practiced here in the late 1960s and early 1970s.

The pioneering spirit is strong at The Chicago Lighthouse, and our clinic has evolved into the world-class Sandy and Rick Forsythe Center for Comprehensive Vision Care, which was dedicated in the fall of 2010. This center has a model system of care that includes specialists in medical retina, low vision optometry, vision rehabilitation research, adaptive technology, occupational therapy, and rehabilitation counseling, and the Bergman Institute for Psychological Support, as its core resources, all under one roof. The integration of these programs allows for total care of the patient, from a diagnosis, to prescribing the most relevant optical devices and training patients to use them, to psychological and employment counseling where we aim to help patients achieve their goals. Within these programs, we investigate new treatment protocols and methods and, in this way, advance the field of vision rehabilitation. These components have training programs where students have the opportunity to learn about the model, and subsequent generations of practitioners can become fluent in the method.

OUT OF SIGHT: A PARTNERSHIP

It was Lindy Bergman's interest in The Lighthouse and our plans for this all-inclusive template for care that brought us together. Lindy, having dealt with her own emotional struggles with AMD, was interested in helping others learn how to cope. She introduced The Chicago Lighthouse clinical staff to the first edition of her book, *Out of Sight, Not Out of Mind,* and it was an immediate hit. Our staff felt that it was a book that was needed to help patients understand that they are not alone. We felt that it could be enormously beneficial for the patient to have Lindy's perspective combined with information from professionals. The concept for the book developed as a resource that would enable patients to become fully informed about their condition. There was a consensus that a disconnect existed between all of the resources available to patients and the patient's ability to benefit from these resources. Also, it was unanimously agreed that the field was in need of a book to help practitioners to understand that their patients required care not only for their eyes, but for their minds as well.

This second edition of *Out of Sight, Not Out of Mind* represents a natural partnership that grew out of the life experiences of Lindy and the professional staff at The Lighthouse. The book reflects our contemporary practice model of what we believe to be the best care that can be offered to patients faced with AMD, or any progressive retinal degenerative disease. It also communicates a standard that we hope will be more commonly learned and adopted by eye care practitioners and rehabilitation centers across the country and throughout the world. We envision that it will become rare for patients to have to search out doctors and piece together a program of care that includes the essential components, as they must do now in many places.

In Part 2 of this book, you will hear from Gerald Fishman, M.D., a renowned ophthalmologist who specializes in the diagnosis of inherited retinal disease and is a scientific advisor to the Foundation Fighting Blindness. He is the director of our Pangere Center for Inherited Retinal Diseases at The Chicago Lighthouse, which is a major referral center for patients who often have difficult-to-diagnose inherited eye conditions. Alfred Rosenbloom, O.D., who was mentioned earlier and is a member of the American Optometric Association's Hall of Fame, contributes a chapter on the low vision optometric evaluation of patients with various eye diseases.

David Rakofsky, Psy.D., a licensed clinical psychologist who leads our Bergman Institute for Psychological Support, writes about how Lindy's story is not so different from every patient's story. It is the view of a human being who overcomes the most feared of all disabling conditions,[6] through strong will, optimism, and hope. Her hope was provided by a young ophthalmologist who told her that she would never become completely blind.

Kara Crumbliss, O.D., who also specializes in low vision optometry and is director of our low vision clinic, offers her unique approach to low vision rehabilitation and a review of the most effective optical enhancement devices. Tom Perski, M.A., our senior vice president of rehabilitation, who has a juvenile form of macular degeneration known as Stargardt macular dystrophy and is a leader in the field of adaptive technology, reports on new developments in this area.

Patricia Grant, M.S., The Chicago Lighthouse's director of research, provides her perspective on the need for research to develop and evaluate new rehabilitation training strategies. Even though retinal prosthetics, gene therapies, and new optical implants are on the horizon, patients will still be in need of rehabilitation to help them make sense of their newly altered, perhaps fragmented, visual worlds.

It is our feeling that all patients can be provided with hope through accurate information about their disease, and by counsel from the kinds of people who can provide effective help. Lindy's belief is that through this optimism she has coped, and it is what led her to be so passionate about supporting others. We are grateful to Lindy for sharing her personal story with all of us, and for having such a lasting and global impact on the field of vision rehabilitation.

NOTES

1. What Is AMD? Los Angeles: AMD.org: Macular Degeneration Partnership, www.amd.org/what-is-amd.html.

2. David S. Friedman, Benita J. O'Colmain, Beatriz Munoz et al., "Prevalence of Age-Related Macular Degeneration in the United States," *Archives of Ophthalmology* 122, no. 4 (2004): 564–72.

3. Patricia Grant, William Seiple, and Janet Szlyk, "The Impact of Depression on the Actual and Perceived Effects of Reading Rehabilitation for People with Central Vision Loss," *Journal of Rehabilitation Research and Development* 48, no. 9 (2011).

4. Cynthia Owsley, Gerald McGwin, Paul P. Lee, Nicole Wasserman, and Karen Searcey, "Characteristics of Low-Vision Rehabilitation Services in the United States," *Archives of Ophthalmology* 127, no. 5 (2009): 681–89.

5. Elisabeth Kübler-Ross, *On Death and Dying* (London: Routledge, 1969).

6. Key Findings: National Poll on Severe Vision Loss/Blindness, American Foundation for the Blind Senior Site, www.afb.org/seniorsite.asp?SectionID=68&TopicID=320&DocumentID=3376.

CHAPTER 7

Vision and Aging
General and Clinical Perspectives

Alfred A. Rosenbloom, Jr.

Providers of vision rehabilitation services are finding that their patient populations are becoming increasingly older and experiencing visual impairments later in life, rather than from congenital causes. Accordingly, this chapter will focus on important aspects in the provision of comprehensive low vision rehabilitation services for older patients seeking such services.

VISUAL IMPAIRMENT DEFINED

Visual impairment, which can be defined as a vision loss that cannot be corrected to normal by eyeglasses or contact lenses, can be linked to basic aging processes, age-related diseases that indirectly affect vision, and the greater probability of accidents as people live longer. In addition to age, visual impairment may sometimes be linked to gender. It is noteworthy that for the 65-and-over age group, more women than men are affected.

Visual impairment is typically quantified in terms of visual acuity and visual field. *Visual acuity* is the amount of detail a person is able to see and is measured and expressed numerically in comparison to normal vision. A person who has normal vision is said to have 20/20 vision. In this expression, the first number refers to the distance at which the person being tested can see a letter on an eye chart, while the second number is the distance at which a person with normal vision can see the same thing. Thus, for example, an individual with 20/70 acuity can see at a distance of 20 feet what a person with 20/20 vision can see at 70 feet. The larger the second number in the scale, the poorer the vision.

Visual field describes the area that an eye can see when looking straight ahead and is measured as an angle, in degrees. A person with normal vision who is looking straight ahead will be able to see objects in a half-circle, approximately a 180-degree range.

Another classification of vision is *legal blindness*. This category was created to determine which individuals would be eligible for government assistance because of their visual impairment, and it is based on both visual acuity and visual field. A person with 20/200 vision or less in the better eye with best possible correction (that is, someone who can see at 20 feet what a person with normal vision is able to see at 200 feet) is considered *legally blind*. A person is also considered to be legally blind if he or she can see only a 20-degree visual field diameter or less concentrically in the better eye. A deficit in visual field may result in loss of either *central* or *peripheral* (side) vision, or both.

Although legal blindness is still used as a criterion for certain services, it does not necessarily indicate how well a person actually functions with the amount of vision he or she has (which is termed *functional vision*). Thus, a person who is not legally blind according to the visual acuity or visual field measured by an eye care specialist might still be considered visually impaired. When an individual has a visual impairment significant enough to interfere with daily living tasks, the person is said to have *low vision*.

LEADING CAUSES OF VISION LOSS

There are certain changes in the eye and visual function that typically accompany aging and in that sense are considered "normal." They usually do not lead to visual impairment. For example, changes involving sensitivity to glare, a need for increased lighting, decreased color perception, reduced contrast sensitivity, and decreased depth perception often develop as individuals age but are not in themselves considered visual impairments. As already indicated, however, the rate of visual impairment does increase among older people.

The four eye diseases or conditions that are the primary causes of visual impairment in older people are cataracts, diabetic retinopathy, glaucoma, and age-related macular degeneration. It is not unusual for people to experience more than one of these conditions, either consecutively or simultaneously.

Cataracts

Cataract is defined as a painless, progressive clouding of the lens of the eye, the transparent structure that brings light rays into focus (see Figure 7.1). Cataracts are an almost inevitable natural result of aging. The condition may develop asymmetrically between eyes, and the degree of impairment can vary greatly among individuals. Fortunately, most people are not affected to the point of significant visual disability. Cataracts do make people, objects,

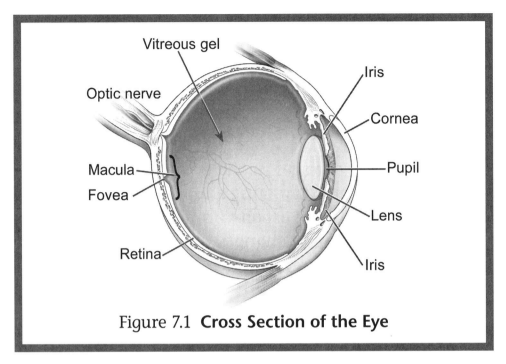

Figure 7.1 **Cross Section of the Eye**

Source: National Eye Institute

and colors appear hazy and "washed out." The lack of detail may make it difficult to read, tell time, watch television, and walk safely, since depth perception may also be affected.

How cataracts are formed is not known. Basically, the opacity that develops in the normally clear lens of the eye is caused by some change in the internal structure of the lens. As lens fibers coagulate, lens protein becomes insoluble and opaque. The treatment for cataracts is removal of the lens. Today, this is a safe surgical procedure that can be performed under local or general anesthesia. The usual procedure, performed by an ophthalmologist, includes removing the clouded lens and, in most cases, replacing it with an *intraocular implant,* or artificial lens. Better vision results in 98 percent of all patients, and the complication rate is low. For those who do not receive intraocular implants, corrective eyeglasses or contact lenses are required.

Diabetic Retinopathy

Diabetic retinopathy is a condition that almost always affects both eyes and appears to some degree in most people who have had diabetes mellitus for at least 10 years. Long-standing diabetes may cause vascular changes that affect the small blood vessels supplying the retina of the eye, the interior layer that reacts to light and transmits visual images through the optic nerve to the brain and other ocular structures (see Figure 7.1; see also Chapter 8 for more information about the retina). Because medical advances can enable diabetes to be better controlled today, many patients live longer, and there is an increased frequency of diabetic retinopathy among individuals with diabetes. If patients follow prescribed regimens carefully, however, particularly in regard to diet and exercise, it seems to lessen the severity of retinal damage. In retinopathy, the actual retinal pathology is seen as microaneurysms, or small hemorrhages, causing scattered "blind spots," known as *scotomas*. Abnormal new blood vessels are also formed that leak fluid and distort vision. Although there is no cure for the retinal disease, laser surgery helps to close new and leaky blood vessels.

Glaucoma

Glaucoma, another serious eye ailment commonly found in older people, is a condition in which elevated *intraocular pressure* (pressure within the eye) results in loss of the visual field and damage to the optic nerve. The *aqueous humor,* a watery fluid located between the cornea and the lens, is formed in the posterior chamber behind the *iris,* the colored portion of the eye, and then circulates through the pupil into the anterior chamber (see Figure 7.2). Here it is drained through the *trabecular meshwork* into the *Canal of Schlemm* at the angle between the rim of

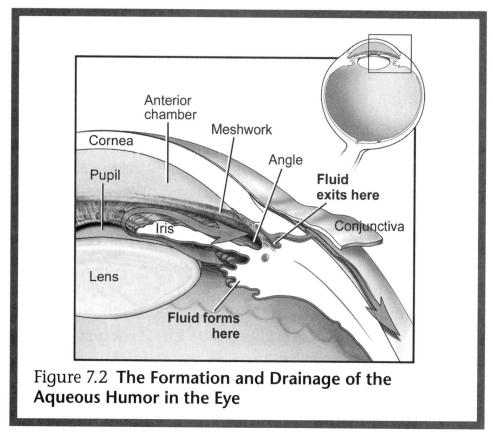

Figure 7.2 **The Formation and Drainage of the Aqueous Humor in the Eye**

Source: National Eye Institute

the iris and the posterior surface of the *cornea,* a transparent protective layer that covers the surface of the eye. The balance between the secretion of this fluid, which nourishes the cornea and the lens, and its outflow determines the intraocular pressure. An increase in pressure can compress blood vessels within the eyeball and thereby deprive the retina of an adequate blood supply, resulting in impaired vision and even blindness.

Treatment usually involves medication to lower intraocular pressure. Pressure generally can be reduced by increasing aqueous outflow with medications that cause the pupil of the eye to contract, or by decreasing the formation of the aqueous fluid with carbonic anhydrase inhibitors or beta-blocking agents. If this treatment fails, a drainage pathway through the trabecular meshwork can be created with laser surgery or by conventional glaucoma surgical techniques.

Macular Degeneration

Age-related macular degeneration is the leading cause of visual impairment among older persons. It can occur at any age but is most common in older people. The symptoms are a progressive loss of central or reading vision and of sharp distance vision, usually in both eyes. As the retina degenerates in this disease, central vision is gradually reduced, even though side vision is maintained. Although the exact cause of this degeneration is unknown, the process is associated with the macular area, the small portion of the retina that includes the fovea, the most sensitive place for acuity within the retina, where the sharpest vision takes place (see Chapter 8 for a detailed discussion of the possible causes and current treatments of AMD).

Low vision devices are the most common method of rehabilitation used for people with macular degeneration. *Low vision devices* are devices that use optical lenses to maximize visual function and may include telescopes, spectacles, or magnifiers in various designs in order to meet specific lifestyle needs. (See Chapters 10 and 11 for discussion of low vision devices and technology.)

CONSEQUENCES OF VISUAL IMPAIRMENT

Demographic aging is a phenomenon of the 20th and 21st centuries. In 1900, 3.1 million people in the United States were age 65 and over, making up about 4.1 percent of the population. By 1980, more than 25 million people were age

65 and over, representing 11.3 percent of the population.[1] In 2010, 40.2 million were in the 65-and-over age group (13 percent of the population), and it is estimated that by 2030, 72 million people will be in this age group.[2]

Given the universality of aging and the increasing number of older persons in society, the causes and consequences of visual changes that accompany age assume greater significance. The decline and selected severe deterioration of vision typically occurs with age, and virtually all persons must adjust to some reduction in visual functioning as they age. Older people often feel the impact of visual impairment more keenly because of other problems associated with aging, such as physical and psychological changes, economic limitations, loss of social independence, and altered roles in the family, the workplace, and the community.

Research has documented the increased prevalence of chronic health conditions among older persons who are visually impaired, including hearing loss, arthritis, high blood pressure, heart conditions, and orthopedic impairments.[3] These impairments are only part of the difficulties visually impaired older people cope with on physical and psychological levels. In addition, the problems commonly associated with the aging process include separation from family members, the loss of a spouse, withdrawal from earlier life roles, retirement, a decrease in overall income, and the loss of family and friends. Not surprisingly, the onset of vision loss exacerbates the other problems associated with attempts to maintain an independent lifestyle.

ADAPTATION TO VISUAL IMPAIRMENT

Often older people with declining visual function can no longer rely on visual cues to compensate for other sensory

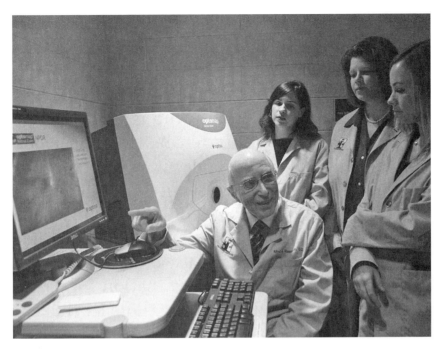

Dr. Rosenbloom and team members. Vision rehabilitation is typically carried out by a team that includes eye care specialists, vision rehabilitation professionals, psychologists, and other allied health care providers. (The Chicago Lighthouse for People Who Are Blind or Visually Impaired)

and physiological losses. Difficulties with mobility associated with vision loss may exacerbate an already unsteady gait and existing balance problems, for example. Moreover, the cumulative stress, anxiety, and depression that often result from these losses may make it more difficult for older people to use their remaining strength and energy.

Overall, there are several mechanisms for coping with vision loss. Other sensory modalities may be used more extensively. In addition, the patient can utilize low vision rehabilitation services designed to provide assessment of visual needs and training in the use of adaptive techniques, which may be provided by a team consisting of an ophthalmologist, optometrist, vision rehabilitation professionals, and other allied health care providers. (For a discussion of low vision rehabilitation, see Chapters 10 and 11.) Social support systems, including the family and close friends, can also be used (see Chapter 9).

A comprehensive low vision examination is an essential service for the older person who is visually impaired (see Chapter 10). Low vision rehabilitation includes not only the prescription of appropriate low vision devices but also instruction and supportive services to enhance the person's performance in the tasks of daily living. Adaptive training involves relearning processes that may include the use of eye movements with the use of low vision devices, determining the appropriate illumination for particular tasks, and developing a modified procedure for the recognition of letters and words.

Various studies have reported a greater than 80 percent success rate in rehabilitating low vision patients who previously were thought to be unable to perform tasks of daily living.[4] Both the team approach and a professional examiner's positive attitude toward low vision rehabilitation are essential contributing factors to success. The team approach typically includes the provision of services by eye care specialists, vision rehabilitation therapists (formerly called rehabilitation teachers), orientation and mobility specialists who specialize in techniques to facilitate independent travel, occupational therapists, psychologists, and social workers.

IMPLICATIONS FOR WORKING WITH OLDER PEOPLE WHO ARE VISUALLY IMPAIRED

Just as each person's visual impairment is unique, so is the individual's reaction to the impairment. Members of the rehabilitation team working with older individuals who are visually impaired should encourage them to become aware of the potential for living more independently by helping them to learn alternative methods of carrying out their everyday activities and desired pursuits and to understand the uncertainties associated with adapting to their visual impairment. The process of rehabilitation, involving adapting, constructing a new environment, and modifying one's self-image, may be uneven and stressful. Given the uncertainties, uneven pace, and stress of the situation, support and rehabilitative services are essential and can provide an important support for more positive outcomes.

The ebb and flow of formulating and reformulating new priorities and goals is an essential part of healthy functioning and adaptation. The professional can assist the person to adjust successfully to visual impairment by being warm and empathetic, having a positive attitude toward the individual, and being realistic in counseling and planning efforts.

Key Principles for Effective Geriatric Patient Care

For rehabilitation professionals working with older individuals, the following principles are a guide to effective care, regardless of the individual's specific condition:

+ Distinguish aging from disease.
+ See the patient as a whole person, focusing on health status, ability, psychosocial well-being, and socioeconomic needs.
+ Use a team approach that includes support resources from the family, community services, health care and

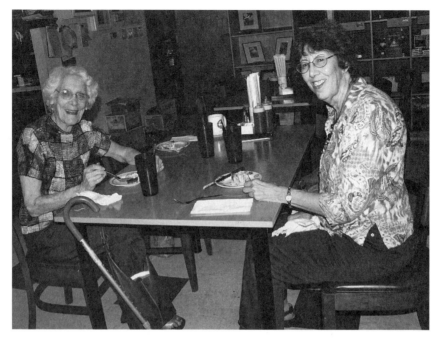

People in later life, including those with AMD, continue to be vibrant, productive members of their families and communities who pursue their interests and activities and live independent lives. (Anne L. Corn)

rehabilitation, social services counseling, and occupational therapy, including environmental support services.

✦ Emphasize the goals of geriatric patient care, including prevention, preservation, restoration, and maintenance, leading to an enhanced quality of life.

✦ Improve the patient's quality of life by facilitating independence and goal-directed activity.

Vision Rehabilitation Therapy

Vision rehabilitation therapy, a key aspect of vision rehabilitation, is defined as "a professional discipline in which instruction and guidance is provided to visually impaired individuals through individualized plans of instruction designed to permit the individuals to carry out their daily activities, to manage their lives more efficiently within their environment, and to reach their potential for self-independence, self-esteem and productivity."[5] In many respects, the profession of vision rehabilitation therapy or rehabilitation teaching reinforces a powerful dimension of the disability movement: the theme of empowerment. By learning skills in communication, activities of daily living, and personal management, individuals are empowered and enabled to carry out the activities that are valuable to them.

People in their later years of life are very much distinct individuals. They have different life histories, personal characteristics, occupations, activities, and preferences. Contrary to the outdated stereotype of frailty and illness in old age, older men and women continue to be vibrant, productive, involved members of their families and communities. They continue to pursue their interests and activities and discover new ones, enjoy increased leisure time, and continue to live independent, dynamic lives. Psychologist G. Stanley Hall, who wrote one of his final pieces, *Senescence: The Last Half of Life,* at age 78, has been described as believing that old age can be seen "not as a period of decline and decay," but rather "as a stage of development in which the passions of youth and the efforts of a life career had reached fruition and consolidation."[6] The use of vision rehabilitation therapy in the face of vision loss can support this dynamic concept of lifetime learning and living.

NOTES

1. Wan He, Manisha Sengupta, Victoria A. Velkoff, and Kimberly A. DeBarros, "65+ in the United States: 2005," *Current Population Reports,* National Institute on Aging and U.S. Census Bureau, 2005, www.census.gov/prod/2006pubs/p23-209.pdf.

2. Lindsay M. Howden and Julie A. Meyer, "Age and Sex Composition: 2010," *2010 Census Briefs*, U.S. Census Bureau, 2011, www.census.gov/prod/cen2010/briefs/c2010br-03.pdf; Grayson K. Vincent and Victoria A. Velkoff, "The Next Four Decades—The Older Population in the United States: 2010 to 2050," *Population Estimates and Projections, Current Population Reports,* U.S. Census Bureau, 2010, www.census.gov/prod/2010pubs/p25-1138.pdf.

3. Alfred A. Rosenbloom, "Prognostic Factors in Low Vision Rehabilitation," *American Journal of Optometry* 47, no. 8 (1970): 600–605. (Note: This pioneering study has not been replicated.) See also John E. Crews, Gwyn C. Jones, and Julie H. Kim, "Double Jeopardy: The Effects of Comorbid Conditions among Older People with Vision Loss," *Journal of Visual Impairment & Blindness* 100, special suppl. (2006): 824–48.

4. Rosenbloom, "Prognostic Factors in Low Vision Rehabilitation."

5. Richard L. Brilliant, ed., *Essentials of Low Vision Practice* (Woburn, MA: Butterworth Heinemann, 1999), 368–72.

6. Tamara K. Hareven, "The Last Stage: Historical Adulthood and Old Age," *Daedalus* 105, no. 4 (1976): 13–27.

CHAPTER 8

Age-Related Macular Degeneration

Causes and Current Medical Perspectives

Gerald Allen Fishman

INTRODUCTORY NOTE

The contents of this chapter are intended to present today's medical perspectives on the important topic of the development of age-related macular degeneration (AMD). They may be best understood by readers who have at least a fundamental knowledge about the human retina and the changes in this structure that can result in AMD. However, an attempt has been made to define various terms that might not be readily understood by the general public. Nonetheless, the topics of retinal anatomy, subtypes of AMD, and various factors responsible for the retinal degeneration that occurs in this disease will require some degree of careful reading. Similarly, sections of the chapter pertaining to various factors that likely contribute to the development of AMD and treatment strategies may require a little patience and persistence on the reader's behalf.

With this in mind, dedication to the task will be rewarded by gaining new and important information that will benefit those experiencing AMD, as well as their family

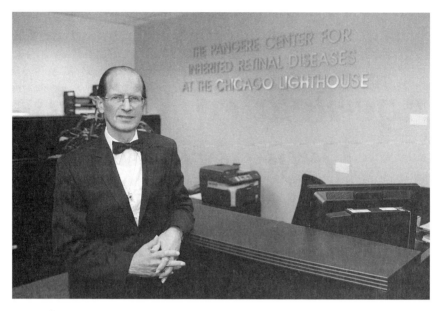

Dr. Fishman at the Pangere Center for Inherited Retinal Diseases at The Chicago Lighthouse. (The Chicago Lighthouse for People Who Are Blind or Visually Impaired)

members. Visual practitioners and trainees, as well as counselors for individuals who are blind or visually impaired, will find information that will be useful for their counseling of patients.

Readers should also note that the chapter is not comprehensively referenced. A selected supplemental list of articles is provided for further reading.

AGE-RELATED MACULAR DEGENERATION: AN OVERVIEW

As our population ages, the need to maintain good visual function becomes a more important factor in the ability of seniors to live happy, productive, and independent lives. The economic cost of visual impairment in the United States totals in the billions of dollars annually, with expenses related to direct medical costs, medical care, and lost productivity each contributing to the total.

Age-related macular degeneration (AMD) has been cited as the third leading cause of legal blindness worldwide and most common cause of legal blindness in industrialized countries (see Chapter 7). This disease has been estimated to affect more than 50 million people worldwide. It is the leading cause of incurable legal blindness in the United States. Some statistics from the United States show that 8 percent of people older than age 65 display an intermediate degree of severity in AMD, while 12 percent of those older than 80 have an advanced form of the disease. Other data have indicated that some degree of AMD affects one in five people over the age of 65 in this country. Also in the United States, an advanced stage of AMD was reported as accounting for 75 percent of legal blindness in adults over age 50.[1] By the year 2020, the prevalence of advanced AMD is estimated to increase by 50 percent. For this reason, attention to modifying behavior as it pertains to reducing risk factors for AMD and both developing new and implementing known evidence-based treatment strategies becomes vital.

Before discussing various aspects of macular degeneration, it is helpful to review basic anatomy of the retina, the inner sensory nerve layer of the eye that plays a central role in the complex processing involved in generating vision by reacting to light and transmitting impulses to the brain. More specifically, it is helpful to understand the central portion of the retina referred to as the macula, which provides our sharpest vision and perception of visual detail. (See the diagram of a cross section of the eye in Chapter 7 for an overview of the anatomy.) The discussion here focuses on those cells or tissues of the macula that are most impaired in AMD.

As just indicated, the term *macula* defines a central region of the retina in which the cone cells of the eye, which are described in the discussion that follows, are most dense and interact with cells further up in the retinal structure in a manner that facilitates our best visual acuity. For reasons yet to be fully identified, this region of the retina is most susceptible to the effects of aging. Some factors considered to contribute to the macula's susceptibility include sustained exposure to light due to its central location within the retina, increased energy demands arising from vigorous metabolic activity set off by this light exposure, high oxygen consumption that accompanies these processes, and the resulting enhanced need for nutrients such as antioxidants.

RETINAL ANATOMY

Although the popular conception of vision is that it is created by the eye, we do not "see" with our eyes, but rather with our brains. Vision results from transmission of electrical energy, which begins in the eye with the conversion of light rays into electrical signals. The retina, a complex structure consisting of several layers that are intimately related, plays a key role in this process, which involves many interactions and functions that affect cell replenishment and survival. (See Figure 8.1 for a diagram of normal retinal structure.)

Photoreceptors: Rods and Cones

The most critical structures directly involved with visual function are the *rods* and *cones*—the *photoreceptor cells*. The term *photoreceptor* refers to their function of absorbing

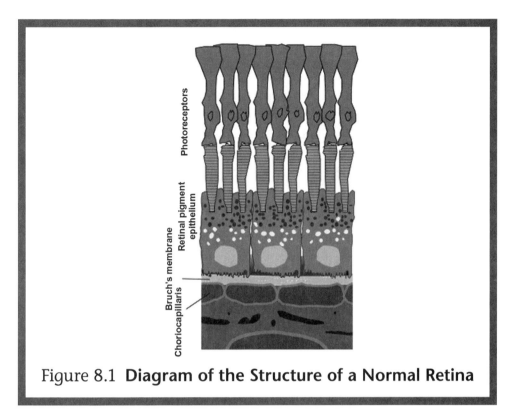

Photoreceptors

Retinal pigment epithelium

Bruch's membrane

Choriocapillaris

Figure 8.1 **Diagram of the Structure of a Normal Retina**

Source: Courtesy of François Delori, 2011

photons, or units of light energy. There are approximately 120–125 million rods and 5–8 million cones in the human retina. Rods function best under dim light, while cones function under brighter illumination and are responsible for our color vision and best visual acuity, the ability to see fine detail. Cones and rods begin the process of vision by absorbing light in a region referred to as *outer segments*. These outer segments are composed of visual pigments that are altered, or "bleached," in their structure when they absorb light of various wavelengths.

When the visual pigments within the rods and cones are altered, the light energy they have absorbed is converted to electrical energy, an electrical signal that in turn is transmitted through the layers of the retina to the optic nerve. From there the visual signal is transmitted to a region of the brain termed the visual cortex, which is housed in the occipital lobe, the very back portion of the brain, where the visual signal is actually interpreted.

Retinal Pigment Epithelium

While deterioration of the rods and cones within the macula directly relates to the poor vision experienced by patients with AMD, there are cells directly underneath the layer of rods and cones, termed the *retinal pigment epithelium* (RPE), which are responsible for sustaining the rods and cones. They supply them with the nutrients they need to survive. When the cells of the RPE degenerate, the photoreceptor cells will also eventually deteriorate from lack of nutritional support. Therefore, normally functioning RPE cells are necessary to sustain rods and cones and, in turn, to help preserve normal visual acuity.

Each day, rods and cones eliminate, or shed, approximately 10 percent of their outer segment length from their region nearest the RPE cells (that is, the distal portion) and resynthesize the same percentage at the opposite (or proximal) end. The shed outer segments, with the vitamin A they contain, are engulfed by the cells of the RPE and are partially digested, in a process referred to as phagocytosis. The vitamin A content of the shed outer segments is initially stored within the RPE cells and then recycled back to the outer segments of the rods and cones for continued maintenance of their structure and function. Without this support from the RPE, the rods and cones could not survive: vitamin A is a vital component of their visual pigments, without which they could not effectively convert light energy into an electrical signal—

the signal that ultimately is interpreted in the brain as a visual experience.

The cells of the retinal pigment epithelium pay a price for their generous support of the photoreceptor cells, the rods and cones. The shed portion of the outer segments is only partially digested by the RPE cells in the process of returning, or recycling, vitamin A to the photoreceptors. The chronic accumulation of outer segment debris leads to the buildup of a waste material termed *lipofuscin* within the RPE cells. Eventually, the accumulation of this material can become toxic to the cells of the RPE and lead to cell death. Damage to these cells affects the transport of nutrients to the photoreceptor cells, which in turn leads to their progressive deterioration. In addition, this damage to the RPE—as well as to its supporting structure, called *Bruch's membrane*— can promote the development of new blood vessels that can leak fluid and blood, resulting in a severe form of AMD, referred to as exudative, or "wet," AMD, with a marked loss of visual function. (Later in this discussion, the roles of light exposure, free radicals, and inflammation will be explained as they relate to the accumulation of lipofuscin.) This destructive relationship is key to the development of more than one form of AMD.

Choroid

A third structure necessary for maintaining normal retinal function is the *choroid*—specifically, the blood vessels in the choroid. This layer of vascular tissue resides underneath the cells of the retinal pigment epithelium. The blood vessels of the choroid (which include the *choriocapillaris*) deliver oxygen to the outer retina, including the RPE and photoreceptor cells. The choroid also assists retinal survival by removing waste material delivered to it by the RPE cells. The choroidal circulation also delivers various nutrients to the RPE and, ultimately, the photoreceptor cells, such as vitamins A and E, as well as zinc, each of which is important for normal functioning of the photo-receptor cells. However, it is also from the choroidal circulation that new blood vessels originate, a process referred to as neovascularization. These new vessels are the source of bleeding into the retina that can occur in patients with one form of AMD.

Bruch's Membrane

Finally, Bruch's membrane, the supporting structure mentioned earlier, can be found between the cells of the retinal pigment epithelium and the choroidal circulation. This membrane serves as a filter or gatekeeper for both nu-trients and unwanted substances that either should or should not gain entrance to the retina. In patients with AMD, this membrane undergoes harmful changes that endanger the health of the rods and cones by depriving them of vital nutrients when waste material accumulates within its structure.

SUBTYPES OF AMD

AMD has been classified into two general types, *non-exudative,* or the "dry" form of AMD, and an *exudative,* or "wet," form. The terms *non-exudative* and *exudative* refer, respectively, to whether there is either no clinical evidence of fluid and/or blood or scar tissue in the macula or, alternatively, the presence of fluid and/or blood, associated with the presence of new blood vessels from the choroidal circulation.

The dry form of AMD is associated with the deposition of a waste material, called *drusen,* under the retinal pigment epithelium onto Bruch's membrane, and the thickening of Bruch's membrane. Although the presence of small drusen does not generally seem to be associated with a loss in visual acuity, the presence of large, overlapping, or confluent drusen, and the presence of RPE cell disturbances, predicts a greater likelihood of the development of a more advanced stage of AMD. In more advanced stages, atrophy of the RPE cells and, often, underlying choroidal blood vessels leads to one or more well-defined circular macular scars, termed *geographic atrophy,* and, often, a marked loss of vision to the level of legal blindness. (Legal blindness, as explained in the previous chapter, is defined as best corrected visual acuity no better than 20/200 in the better-seeing eye.) Other changes in the macula observed in the dry form of AMD include disturbances of the cells of the RPE, including both the clumping (hyperpigmentation) and dropout or loss of pigment (hypopigmentation) of the cells. Over time, the condition of a percentage of patients with the dry form of AMD may evolve into a wet form of the disease.

At an earlier stage of the wet form, patients may show an elevation or a detachment of a small segment of RPE cells within the macular region from the presence of fluid. As the wet form advances, new blood vessels from the choroid initially invade beneath the RPE. These vessels can bleed, causing subsequent scarring within the macula and a loss of RPE and photoreceptor cells, with a resultant severe loss of visual acuity.

Data analysis shows that 80 to 90 percent of patients seen in retinal practices for the evaluation and possible treatment of AMD have various stages of dry AMD, versus

10 to 15 percent with a wet form of this disorder. Additional analysis shows that 3.5 percent of patients over the age of 75 years have the geographic atrophy form of dry AMD and corresponding severe loss of their visual acuity.

DISEASE-CAUSING MECHANISMS

Exposure of the macula to light—particularly to ultra-violet and short wavelength, or blue, light—coupled with high energy demands on the macula, and the resultant high consumption of oxygen, leads to the formation of molecules called *free radicals*. The formation of free radicals results in the destruction of the outer segments of photoreceptor cells, which have an abundant content of lipids, or fats, in their membranes, by a process called *lipid peroxidation*. Peroxidation involves the destruction by high-energy oxygen molecules of lipid membranes that compose the structure of cells such as rods and cones.

The destruction of outer segments of the rods and cones results in an accumulation of debris consisting of these outer segments within the retinal pigment epithelium cells of the macula. As noted earlier, a portion of this photoreceptor debris that cannot be digested by the RPE accumulates within RPE as lipofuscin. A component of lipofuscin is a substance abbreviated as A2E. This substance readily absorbs blue light, which in turn leads to the production of harmful free radicals. In addition, the accumulation of A2E disrupts the process of phagocytosis by which outer segments of the rods and cones are engulfed by the cells of the RPE and the digestion of outer segment membranes. This enhanced accumulation of lipofuscin and A2E leads also to damage of the RPE cells and, consequently, the rods and cones of the retina. In turn, the deterioration of RPE cells stimulates an immune-response-mediated chronic inflammation, which is governed by a process referred to as the *complement system.*

The complement process is part of the normal immune system. It can potentially play a protective role vis-à-vis disease by generating several factors that facilitate the destruction of foreign organisms and abnormal cells. In certain instances, however, activation of the complement system further contributes to the local damage of the retinal pigment epithelium and photoreceptor cells, the thickening of Bruch's membrane, and the formation of drusen, as well as choroidal neovascularization, followed by fluid and hemorrhagic, or bleeding, changes in the macula, with resultant visual loss. Abnormal activation of the complement system will be discussed under the next section on risk factors.

RISK FACTORS

Conclusions drawn from primarily epidemiological studies have provided evidence for the association of family history, advanced age, genetics, smoking history, use of alcohol, consumption of saturated and omega-6 fatty acids, systemic hypertension, atherosclerotic cardiovascular disease, and exposure to ultraviolet and blue light from sunlight exposure with an increased risk for the development of AMD.[2] In contrast, dietary factors such as lutein and zeaxanthin, present in green leafy vegetables, and in most studies omega-3 fatty acids, enriched in fish, are associated with a reduced risk for the development of AMD.[3] A national clinical study with the use of vitamin supplements and the mineral zinc (discussed later in this chapter in the section on treatment strategies) has shown these substances to be of some modest but statistically significant value in reducing the incidence of a more advanced form of AMD in some patients. These various dietary factors may be of value by either neutralizing the harmful effect of free radicals or possibly reducing their formation.

Epidemiological studies have implicated genetic factors that influence the development of AMD to the extent that family members of those experiencing the condition are potentially at increased risk of developing the disease.[4] Findings from studies involving both families and twins support the existence of a genetic component in the development of AMD.[5]

A genetic variation in the factor H gene related to the complement system (the CFH gene) has been associated with a higher frequency of the development of AMD. This mutation, termed Y402H, results in the amino acid substitution of a histidine for tyrosine at the amino acid position 402 of the complement protein. Fifty percent of AMD patients will show the Y402H variant of CFH as compared to 29 percent of non-AMD patients. This mutation in factor H releases its usual control over the development of inflammation, resulting in an increased inflammatory response. The modified genetic form of CFH has been identified in the development of a high-risk form of "soft," or less sharply defined, drusen and advanced forms of AMD. In addition, inherited genetic variations involving other complement system factors such as complement factor 3 (C3), complement factor B (CFB), complement factor I (CFI), and complement H-related 1 and 3 genes, were each shown to be significant risk factors for AMD.

TREATMENT STRATEGIES FOR PATIENTS WITH AMD

In the treatment of AMD, a number of strategies have been established as meaningful ways of managing patients, such as photocoagulation and use of anti-VEGF (vascular endo-thelial growth factor) antibodies. Others, such as platelet-derived growth factor, are in the process of undergoing evaluation in use with patients.

Exudative AMD

Laser Photocoagulation

Laser photocoagulation is an often-used initial ther-apy for the treatment of choroidal neovascularization (CNV) in patients with the exudative, or wet, form of AMD. This mode of treatment is based on the principle that the expo-sure of new blood vessels to high-energy light results in their closure from heat generated by absorption of the laser beam, which reduces or eliminates the leakage of fluid or blood. Various strategies can be used, including intravenous injection of a sensitizing dye prior to use of the laser. The photosensitizing dye has an affinity for the new blood vessels, and the laser beam is more readily ab-sorbed by the dye within the walls of these new vessels. Since the laser-generated heat is more confined to the new vessels, less damage occurs to surrounding, more normal, retinal tissue. Closure of the new blood vessels originating from the choroidal circulation beneath the retina can stop them from growing further, leaking fluid, or bleeding. A scar will form in the retina from the laser treatment that creates a permanent localized blind spot in the treated area.

Laser treatment, when successful, is often only a means for temporarily preventing further loss of vision that often will occur without the use of therapy. In spite of laser treatment, vision may continue to decrease, and laser treatment may be effective in only about 50 percent of treated cases. Even when the laser treatment is initially considered to be successful, new or recurrence of CNV growth can occur months to years later, resulting in further loss of vision.

Treatment Substances

VEGF Inhibitors. Vascular endothelial growth factor, or VEGF, is a protein produced in the retina that promotes vascular leakage of fluid and the development of new blood vessels, referred to as angiogenesis. (The term *angiogenesis* refers to the process of developing new blood vessels; *neovascularization* refers to the blood vessels themselves.) The injection of VEGF inhibitors, such as Lucentis (ranibizumab) or Avastin (bevacizumab), into the vitreous of the eye can improve visual acuity in many patients with neovascular AMD. The vitreous is a liquid substance that fills the eye behind the lens and in front of the retina, which maintains the eye's structure. These drugs control the development of new blood vessels and leakage of fluid from retinal vessels. In most patients, choroidal neovascularization is stabilized but does not generally decrease or regress. In one study with the use of Lucentis, CNV regressed in 16 percent of patients, but in most instances (68 percent of eyes), the neovascularization remained stable. In some patients it progressed. In certain cases, patients require continued monthly dosing of anti-VEGF drugs in order to maintain a beneficial therapeutic effect.[6]

VEGF Trap. VEGF Trap is a VEGF receptor protein in blood vessels that binds all forms of VEGF-A. Given by injection into the vitreous, it can reduce the size of CNV and improve visual acuity.

PDGF Inhibitor. Platelet-derived growth factor (PDGF) is a protein that regulates the growth of cells and is involved with angiogenesis. A PDGF inhibitor was used in combination with the VEGF inhibitor Lucentis as a treatment in 22 patients with CNV. A partial regression of CNV occurred in 91 percent of the patients, while none experienced progression of their CNV. Stabilization of the CNV occurred in 9 percent of eyes.

Sirolimus. A substance called sirolimus has been used in the prevention of rejection of transplanted organs; in coronary artery restenosis, or blockage; and in the treatment of advanced kidney cell cancer. It can inhibit inflammation; the proliferation of cells, including the development of new blood vessels; and the leakage of fluid from blood vessels. In the eye it can be delivered either into the vitreous or below superficial tissue in the front part of the eye called the conjunctiva. Sirolimus can decrease the production of VEGF, reducing leakage of fluid from blood vessels and inhibiting the further growth of CNV. However, caution is warranted with the oral or intravenous use of sirolimus in particular, as there is an issue of potential harmful effects from suppression of the immune system.

Ionizing Radiation

The use of radiation has been considered as a means of treating CNV. Its mechanism of action is through its effect on the endothelial cells that line or coat the inside of blood vessels. It inhibits angiogenesis, diminishing inflammation and inhibiting scar formation associated with CNV.

Small Interfering RNA (SiRNA)

Ribonucleic acid (RNA) is genetic material that translates genetic information coded within deoxynucleic acid (DNA) molecules into protein products. Small interfering RNA, or SiRNA, is a class of RNA molecules that can interfere with the expression of specific genes involved in the development of AMD by interfering with the expression of a genetic code carried by RNA. Using a single intravitreal injection of SiRNA in 27 patients with neovascular AMD, almost 90 percent of these patients showed a stabilization of their visual acuity, while 11 percent of patients showed an improvement of being able to perceive 15 or more additional letters—the equivalent of three additional lines—on an ETDRS (Early Treatment Diabetic Research Study) vision chart. Additional investigations are being planned with the use of repeated administration of SiRNA.

Non-Exudative AMD

Use of Pharmacological Agents

As noted earlier in this chapter, oxidative stress from high-energy oxygen molecules and insufficient levels of micronutrients available to the retina are considered to be important contributory factors for the disease progression in AMD patients. This view assumes that AMD is, at least in part, caused by a lifelong exposure to free radicals that are a by-product of a high level of oxygen consumption in the photoreceptor and retinal pigment epithelium cells of the macula. Other contributing factors were described in the section on risk factors associated with the development of AMD. As explained in the discussion on disease-causing mechanisms contributing to the development of AMD, various factors are in all likelihood responsible for the death of photoreceptor cells and the accumulation of cellular debris within the retina. This debris includes primarily oxidized lipids from deteriorating lipid membranes of the photoreceptor cells. The oxidized lipid membranes, in turn, promote the development of inflammation and possibly cause a direct toxic effect on macular tissues, resulting in AMD.

The Age-Related Eye Disease Study (AREDS)[7] evaluated the effect of substantial doses of vitamins C (500 mg) and E (400 IU), in addition to beta-carotene (15 mg) and zinc (80 mg), on the rate of progression to advanced AMD and on visual acuity. These substances were considered to possibly exert a positive effect on AMD, from their capacity to serve as antioxidants, and reduce the harmful effects of free radicals on the rod and cone photoreceptor cells.

Data from the AREDS study showed a rather limited efficacy of the antioxidant and zinc supplements in individuals with a moderate degree of AMD. A 23 percent rate of progression to an advanced form of AMD was observed in the treatment group, and 28 percent in the control group. In addition, 23 percent of eyes that received treatment showed a 15-letter decrease, equivalent to three lines on an ETDRS vision chart, despite treatment. The current AREDS formulation of nutrients containing beta-carotene is not recommended for smokers, who show a greater risk for developing lung cancer with the use of this formulation. For those individuals with a mild degree of AMD, the benefits of the AREDS supplementation are unproven, and thus it is likely that these supplements should not be recommended for this group of AMD patients. Based on the study's design and methods for data analysis, controversy exists as to the interpretation of the results.[8]

In the AREDS2 follow-up study (see www.areds2.org), the efficacy of what are termed xanthophylls, which include lutein and zeaxanthin, and the role of two omega-3 long-chain polyunsaturated fatty acids, abbreviated DHA and EPA, as well as alpha-linoleic acid, are being evaluated as antioxidants and anti-inflammatory agents for their possible beneficial effects on the progression to advanced forms of AMD. In ongoing evaluations, the elimination of beta-carotene and the reduction of zinc from 80 mg to 25 mg is being tested in AMD patients.

Implant of Cells That Secrete CNTF

Ciliary neurotrophic factor (CNTF) is a substance that has been shown in animals to increase thickness of the retina, particularly the outer nuclear layer of the photoreceptor cells, which might indicate a favorable response. An initial trial of encapsulated retinal pigment cells, genetically modified to produce CNTF, implanted in the vitreous has been in progress. The interpretation of initial results was unclear as to the true efficacy of CNTF in patients with dry AMD.

Fenretinide

Fenretinide is a synthetic substance that binds to retinol-binding protein, a protein that transports vitamin A in the circulation to various tissues of the body. By its binding to retinol-binding protein, fenretinide prevents the uptake of retinol or vitamin A by the retinal pigment epithelium cells, and therefore the amount of vitamin A available to the retina. This in turn can decrease the amount of toxic A2E and lipofuscin accumulation in the RPE, which could be potentially beneficial to patients with a dry form of AMD. Investigation of the use of fenretinide in AMD is in progress. Since this drug slows the recovery of rod function after exposure to light, its use can lead to difficulty adjusting when changing from a light to a dark environment.

Suppression of Inflammation

The role of inflammation in AMD was described previously in the discussion of disease-causing mechanisms, as was the relevance of a mutation in the CFH gene in the section on risk factors associated with AMD. The complement process encompasses a system of serum proteins that are an important component of the human immune system. Inhibition of complement activation might be a reasonable treatment strategy for AMD. A substance termed POT-4 inhibits the activation of complement component 3 and thus might theoretically serve as a benefit for visual function in patients with dry AMD.

A note of caution is warranted, however, when considering therapy that involves a suppression of the complement system, since this system plays a vital role in the defense mechanisms not only in the eye but also throughout the entire body. Therapies that are aimed at suppressing the complement system could result in potentially serious systemic or generalized side effects. Treatments that focus on selectively suppressing potentially harmful variants of complement might be a more prudent treatment strategy.

SUMMARY

From the perspective of a patient with AMD, the goals of treatment would emphasize preventing a dry form of AMD from progressing to the wet form, in which a greater loss of vision is likely to occur. Overall goals would include the preservation of visual acuity or reduction in the rate of its loss; reducing the size of a central scotoma or blind spot, where vision is impaired, or decreasing its rate of progression; and improving reading speed. In addition, more sensitive, noninvasive diagnostic tests that could also serve as prognostic indicators for future disease progression are needed.

Age-related macular degeneration is a complex disease having both genetic and environmental factors that contribute to its development. While AMD almost never causes total blindness, its toll on vision for senior members of society is appreciable. As such, a better understanding of those factors that lead to its development is urgent.

Current research supports the conclusion that the prevention or reduction of oxidative stress, resulting from the formation of high-energy oxygen molecules, and the suppression of inflammation, as well as the means for preserving photoreceptor and retinal pigment epithelium cells, are key areas that warrant emphasis. Also, even more effective means of preventing the development of choroidal neovascularization, and its treatment once it occurs, need to be developed.

Considerable progress in our understanding and treatment of this disease has occurred in the last decade because of a more thorough knowledge of the various factors that lead to degeneration of the photoreceptor cells in patients who develop AMD. As our knowledge continues to deepen, it is likely that even more effective and longer-acting treatment strategies will emerge. Hope is on the horizon. The best is yet to come.

NOTES

1. Ronald Klein, Qin Wang, Barbara E. K. Klein, Scott E. Moss, Stacy M. Meuer, "The Relationship of Age-Related Maculopathy, Cataract, and Glaucoma to Visual Acuity," *Investigative Ophthalmology and Visual Science* 36, no. 1 (1995): 182–91.

2. Kristin K. Snow and Johanna M. Seddon, "Do Age-Related Macular Degeneration and Cardiovascular Disease Share Common Antecedents?," *Ophthalmic Epidemiology* 6, no. 2 (1999): 125–43; Johanna M. Seddon, Sarah George, and Bernard Rosner, "Cigarette Smoking, Fish Consumption, Omega-3 Fatty Acid Intake, and Associations with Age-Related Macular Degeneration: The U.S. Twin Study of Age-Related Macular Degeneration," *Archives of Ophthalmology* 124, no. 7 (2006): 995–1001; Johanna M. Seddon, Bernard Rosner, Robert D. Sperduto, Lawrence Yannuzzi, Julia A. Haller, Norman P. Blair, and Walter Willett, "Dietary Fat and Risk for Advanced Age-Related Macular Degeneration," *Archives of Ophthalmology* 119, no. 8 (2001): 1191–99.

3. Seddon et al., "Cigarette Smoking, Fish Consumption, Omega-3 Fatty Acid Intake"; Johanna M. Seddon, Jennifer Cote, and Bernard Rosner, "Progression of Age-Related Macular Degeneration: Association with Dietary Fat, Transunsaturated Fat, Nuts, and Fish Intake," *Archives of Ophthalmology* 121, no. 12 (2003): 1728–37.

4. Wayne Smith and Paul Mitchell, "Family History and Age-Related Maculopathy: The Blue Mountains Eye Study," *Australian New Zealand Journal of Ophthalmology* 26, no. 3 (1998): 203–6; Leslie Hyman and Rebecca Neborsky, "Risk Factors for Age-Related Macular Degeneration: An Update," *Current Opinion in Ophthalmology* 13, no. 3 (2002): 171–75.

5. Sanford M. Meyers, "A Twin Study of Age-Related Macular Degeneration," *Transactions of the American Ophthalmological Society*

92 (1994): 775–843; Michael L. Klein and Peter J. Francis," Genetics of Age-Related Macular Degeneration," *Ophthalmology Clinics of North America* 16, no. 4 (2003): 567–74.

6. Jason S. Slakter, "What to Do When Anti-VEGF Therapy 'Fails,'" *Retinal Physician* 7 (2010): 35–40.

7. Age-Related Eye Disease Study Research Group, "A Randomized Placebo-Controlled Clinical Trial of High-Dose Supplementation with Vitamins C and E, Beta Carotene, and Zinc for Age-Related Macular Degeneration and Vision Loss," AREDS Report No. 8, *Archives of Ophthalmology* 119, no. 10 (2001): 1417–36.

8. Lee M. Jampol, "Antioxidants, Zinc, and Age-Related Macular Degeneration: Results and Recommendations," *Archives of Ophthalmology* 119, no. 10 (2001): 1533–34.

RECOMMENDED SUPPLEMENTAL READING

David M. Brown, Peter K. Kaiser, Mark Michels, Gisele Soubrane, Jeffrey S. Heier, Robert Y. Kim, Judy P. Sy, and Susan Schneider. "Ranibizumab versus Vereporfin for Neovascular Age-Related Macular Degeneration." *New England Journal of Medicine* 355 (October 5, 2006): 1432–44.

Philip J. Rosenfeld, David M. Brown, Jeffrey S. Heier, David S. Boyer, Peter K. Kaiser, Carol Y. Chung, and Robert Y. Kim. "Ranibizumab for Neovascular Age-Related Macular Degeneration." *New England Journal of Medicine* 355 (October 5, 2006): 1419–31.

Johanna M. Seddon, Umed A. Ajani, and Braxton D. Mitchell. "Familial Aggregation of Age-Related Maculopathy." *American Journal of Ophthalmology* 123, no. 2 (1997): 199–206.

CHAPTER 9

Emotional and Psychological Reactions to Age-Related Macular Degeneration

David M. C. Rakofsky

Previous chapters have described the prevalence and development of age-related macular degeneration and have touched on its potentially devastating impact on the individual's central vision. However, macular degeneration may affect far more than someone's ability to see and to carry out the various activities of everyday living that most of us take for granted. Its progression may be accompanied by a range of emotional and psychological reactions that are commonly experienced by those undergoing significant vision loss.

This chapter outlines these reactions and potential influence on the lives of persons who have age-related macular degeneration, explains the importance of addressing their effects as part of a comprehensive vision rehabilitation program, and describes the psychological support program developed at The Chicago Lighthouse to integrate this critical area of concern into effective treatment for those receiving low vision services.

INITIAL RESPONSE TO VISION LOSS

A diagnosis of age-related macular degeneration is, for the individual, a turning point in life. Activities once taken for granted and performed without thinking may become threatened with disruption, often provoking a range of emotional reactions, from shock to worry to terror and dread. Although people struggling to find their way as vision dims may exhibit symptoms of depression, most of them would not meet criteria for a diagnosis of major depression. Instead, they might experience only a persistent, low-level "subthreshold" depression,[1] which could be described as a cluster of related emotional and physiological symptoms with some troubling aspects of depression that do not on their own meet the criteria for major depression, as described by the American Psychiatric Association.[2]

At various points in the progression of their loss of visual acuity, people may struggle with:

+ diminished self-esteem
+ sadness
+ feelings of hopelessness and helplessness
+ negative ideas about the future
+ listlessness
+ poor appetite
+ problems initiating sleep or staying asleep
+ a lack of interest in things they once enjoyed

Though these feelings are usually not permanent, they nevertheless are reactions worthy of further clinical attention: to help distinguish this response from a major depressive episode, which at its worst can end in suicidal thoughts or, tragically, with actions to end one's life in the most extreme cases.

These emotional and psychosocial reactions to visual impairment are often not taken into consideration during the vision rehabilitation process.[3] (See Chapter 12 for additional discussion of research on psychosocial factors related to vision loss.) A first step in helping a patient engage in low vision rehabilitation with the most promising outcome is to screen for the presence of maladjustment in the first place.[4] The following sections describe the approach used at The Chicago Lighthouse for assessing and treating the commonly found emotional components of vision loss as part of comprehensive treatment.

THE BERGMAN INSTITUTE

Established in October 2008, the Bergman Institute for Psychological Support at The Chicago Lighthouse is one of the world's first full-fledged programs dedicated to psychological support in a low vision clinic, employing clinical psychologists and training future psychologists in the specialty we call "low vision psychology." Low vision psychology is a subdiscipline within the field of psychology at large, emphasizing the treatment and research related to the experience of blindness and vision loss.

The focus of the Bergman Institute is the emotional and psychosocial components of vision loss and their impact on the person's ability to engage in rehabilitative and adjustment efforts. Thus, everything from early-term mood and emotional adjustment screenings in the clinic to research into the prevalence of and best treatments for

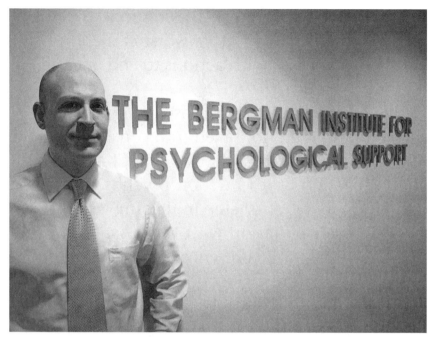

Dr. Rakofsky at the Bergman Institute for Psychological Support at The Chicago Lighthouse. (The Chicago Lighthouse for People Who Are Blind or Visually Impaired)

common mood and morale effects associated with vision loss is within the institute's purview.

Here at the institute, a range of options is offered to people at various stages of vision loss. Options include group therapy, individual and family therapy, psychodiagnostic assessment (which could include personality and/or neuropsychological testing when indicated by a specific referral to the institute or by some significant finding during examination); and brief mandatory psychosocial screenings for all new patients in the low vision clinic of The Lighthouse, as well as for returning patients.

PROTOCOL FOR CARE AND TREATMENT

The typical procedure for a person who has been referred to the institute by another professional (or, just as likely, a person who has elected on his or her own to find out how we can help) is to schedule an appointment by telephone for an assessment. Then we and the patient decide together, in person, whether or not our services (such as individual or, in many cases, group therapy) should be scheduled for a future date. Depending on the level of severity of symptoms experienced, a typical treatment episode can last weeks or months, usually at a weekly pace, and for one-hour sessions. Formal treatment is usually discontinued once the patient experiences sufficient relief and wishes to either stop or wants to attempt taking a break. Treatment may then continue episodically throughout a longer period of adjustment to come.

Each case can be, and usually is, vastly different from any other. In the case of the psychosocial screening protocol that all new patients in the low vision clinic undergo, most established patients meet with us briefly, about once a year before an annual low vision eye exam, and do fine in the interim. They know, of course, that they can call the institute if their morale should take a turn for the worse. While the majority of patients never go into formal therapy with us, we nevertheless believe that meeting members of our staff during regularly scheduled eye exams helps to foster an awareness of our presence in this medical environment, and an awareness of one's need to stay vigilant for signs of an emotional downturn over the course of the vision loss and rehabilitation process. The perception of easy access to what we offer may make the difference between a patient getting professional help when needed and suffering unnecessarily without it.

PSYCHOSOCIAL SCREENING

During the psychosocial screening, undertaken at the beginning of the comprehensive low vision examination visit, psychologists and their supervised trainees may encourage family members who accompany patients to be a part of this brief interview that is a component of the day's activities. (A sample section from this screening is presented in "Sample Questions from The Chicago Lighthouse Psychosocial Screening Interview.") The screening, usually 30 minutes long, is a blend of questions related to how patients are functioning at home and in the community, and an evaluation of how they are handling whatever emotional responses to loss of vision and the threat to independence that they may be experiencing. This step assists the low vision clinic's treatment team members (including optometrists and occupational therapists) who will subsequently work with the patient throughout their treatment. The screening also indicates areas of difficulty in functioning as well as the patient's readiness for any given rehabilitation strategy prescribed.

A specific section of the assessment attempts to identify some fears commonly reported by patients about living with an acquired and progressive eye condition, including fears about being taken advantage of due to decreased vision, fears of being a "burden" to family, and—the most commonly observed fear asked about in the screening—that of losing remaining vision.

Although staff strive to balance issues of privacy with the need to accumulate the most reliable and useful data relating to patients through the screening process, the general conclusion is that having a close relative or trusted friend present for the psychosocial screening is usually more

Sample Questions from The Chicago Lighthouse Psychosocial Screening Interview

The following sample is from the psychosocial interview form used at The Chicago Lighthouse's Bergman Institute for Psychological Support. This particular section focuses on adjustment and recreation.

ADJUSTMENT/RECREATION

It is fairly common for people adjusting to visual loss to experience emotional reactions. Are you experiencing any of the following?

____Frustration; ____Sadness; ____Hopelessness

____Problems with appetite; ____Problems with sleeping

____Restlessness; ____Feeling wound-up, hyper, or nervous?

____Increased feeling of fear in general?

____A fear of being taken advantage of by others?

____A fear of being a burden to your family?

____A fear of losing your remaining vision?

____Other_____

____None

What types of recreational activities do you enjoy?

_____
_____
_____

Has your vision loss impacted your ability to engage in these activities?

_____Yes   _____No

helpful than not. The Lighthouse staff see with some frequency that patients underreport or downplay their real limitations and feel discouragement, even depressive symptoms. Frequently a spouse, daughter, or sibling will nod emphatically to the interviewer in response to certain questions, out of their loved one's line of sight, indicating that the patient is not providing a completely realistic appraisal of the situation. Such nonverbal assistance by family can prove vital in providing the most appropriate treatment plan for some of our more reluctant but needy patients.

In cases in which the individual appears from the interview to be significantly lacking in emotional readiness for the rehabilitation effort to begin, he or she is offered a more thorough and focused assessment. The aim is to see if the patient requires some ongoing or even pre-rehabilitation counseling services to help ready him or her for the process of rehabilitation following the low vision examination. Some patients may report experiencing strange visual hallucinations, discussed in "Charles Bonnet Syndrome: A Rare Psychological Phenomenon."

The more in-depth interview will likely take place on a future date or, in some cases, on the same day that such emotional reactions are being discovered. The additional assessment is offered because it is known from published studies and anecdotal observation alike that rehabilitation outcomes hinge upon psychological adjustment and attitudes about vision loss.[5] Specifically, people who feel that rehabilitation is going to be useless will often experience depressive symptoms and may tend to gain less from efforts to teach them strategies for independent living and adaptation to devices and technologies designed to compensate for lost vision.

Charles Bonnet Syndrome:
A Rare Psychological Phenomenon

From time to time, we hear concerns from our patients with macular degeneration about the spontaneous onset of visual hallucinations in the absence of any history of psychotic symptoms. These same people are very much aware that this is highly unusual for them and that the things they "see" are not actually present, but often visual memories, sometimes personal, such as familiar faces, and other times, patterns and shapes. The images are often highly vivid, complex, and repetitive. The one thing all these people have in common is the fearful question, "Am I going crazy?"

These patients were hardly "losing their minds" but rather are experiencing a neurological event, known as Charles Bonnet Syndrome. There are estimates that about 17 percent of all people with significant acquired central vision loss, such as macular degeneration, will experience this syndrome at some point,[6] for what may range from a few seconds to the majority of the waking day. More recent studies[7] suggest the prevalence may be closer estimated at between 40 and 60 percent.

Simplified greatly, the following is a way to understand how such an event could happen to otherwise mentally healthy older adults. The human brain has areas dedicated to the processing of images. Specifically, electrical signals emanate from an otherwise healthy and functioning retina (the area of the eye upon which focused light is projected) and translate into impulses that are then transmitted to the brain through the optic nerve and visual pathways for both basic and highly sophisticated analysis. In progressed cases of retinal disease such as macular degeneration, there eventually can be an almost absolute lack of "signal" or images of any kind being sent down those visual pathways. What the brain then does with this lack of data or input, this absence of familiar shapes, contours, and colors, is to essentially pull out old memories of

(continued)

Charles Bonnet Syndrome (*continued*)

things seen during the healthier life of the eye and visual system—that includes those intact nervous pathways and the brain's visual processing areas—much like one might start pulling files out of a large library of folders, but in no particular order. The result is an unpredictable course of exclusively visual hallucinations born of sensory deprivation, which could last anywhere from days to years,[8] and which can be manifested as static or animated shapes or faces, most of which are appropriate to the environment as opposed to the bizarre hallucinations found in more psychopathologic conditions, such as schizophrenia. People, sometimes in miniature form, animals, architecture, and outdoor scenes seem to comprise the bulk of descriptions by patients experiencing this usually benign and eventually well-tolerated syndrome of perception.

There are a few important points we make sure to pass on to any patients reporting this condition in an attempt to give them the most useful information toward regaining their emotional equilibrium again, especially since, for so many people, the phenomenon has been a private affair, kept secret from those around them for fear of being thought of as "crazy," with the stigma that flows from that label:

♦ Although we understand that this novel and bizarre experience has the potential to make anyone feel afraid or depressed and to affect daily functioning, understand that the experience has nothing at all to do with a mental condition or emotional disturbance, per se.
♦ "This too shall pass." Charles Bonnet Syndrome is known to cease, usually within 12 to 18 months, and can remit as spontaneously as it first appeared.
♦ There is no treatment for the condition, but just knowing that it is neither an indication of diminishing mental health nor a permanent aspect of your life will likely help you to feel more at ease about it.

✦ Closing your eyes and blinking has been reported to help stop a hallucinatory event,[9] and you may find other reliable ways of temporarily discontinuing a Charles Bonnet event if you try.

✦ "You are not alone." Many others have dealt with this syndrome before you.

It is important to let your primary vision care professional know about the possible presence of any hallucinations right away; distinguishing this condition from a more serious neurological or emotional problem is best done by an eye care professional.

KÜBLER-ROSS'S STAGES OF GRIEF

Institute staff have often noticed impressive correspondence between how people absorb and deal with the bad news of a low vision diagnosis over time and the stages of grief proposed by Elisabeth Kübler-Ross after extensive experience and her study of hundreds of people struggling to cope with a terminal illness and facing death.[10] Kübler-Ross described the stages of grief when facing death as consisting of five principal points that begin with "denial" and progress until the ultimate "acceptance" of what is inevitable for the person undergoing the loss. Generally speaking, once a person has moved out of the initial temporary phase of *denial,* in which the person simply cannot believe that such unfortunate circumstances have befallen him or her, he or she may shift into *anger,* a stage that, in the Kübler-Ross model, can build an emotional distance between the patient and those caring for him or her, including professionals and loved ones alike. This shift is hypothesized to be a manifestation of the rage of being singled out with an affliction, turned outward at the world.

Kübler-Ross called the next stage *bargaining,* in which the patient is struggling with his or her imminent and premature demise and takes part in a kind of internal negotiation for "more time," sometimes in highly irrational and unlikely ways. *Depression,* the stage that she posited follows, is marked by grieving in a way that the person had previously not really engaged in, or not in a manner as focused, intense, or singularly as in this stage. The observable signs of this stage are similar to the symptoms of clinical depression (such as sadness, despondence, negativity in outlook, and isolation), hence the name Kübler-Ross attributed to this penultimate phase of grief. Finally, in *acceptance,* the dying individual comes to terms with mortality, and the preparation for letting go and saying goodbyes is fully initiated, but often in a manner reflecting a peace that the person has made with the inevitable end to his or her earthly existence.

Kübler-Ross herself cautioned that these stages do not necessarily conform to any particular or strictly linear sequence, that they are not complete, and that it is not necessary for one to travel through it in its entirety. Having acknowledged that, however, low vision health care professionals at The Lighthouse have indeed observed patients "stuck" in a stage of denial, bargaining, or anger and depression, only to finally emerge at a point of acceptance of about their vision problems, and ready for rehabilitation, analogous in striking ways to what Kübler-Ross had observed in those dealing with death. It is an aspect of true acceptance, once it is achieved, that people then actively engage in rehabilitation and do not simply reach a kind of blasé resignation or recognition that their vision loss is permanent.

What can make the psychological support of older persons with macular degeneration complicated, however, is the reality that vision can and usually does plateau (that is, seems to reach a point of stasis and stability) only to suddenly deteriorate further in the future. This often requires a new journey through the previously described stages of denial to acceptance. It is the belief of the institute's treatment staff that through an episode of effective psychological intervention, patients can become more resilient in the face of upcoming diminutions of their vision over time, rather than simply being destined to suffer equally with each new setback.

CRISES OF IDENTITY

People with progressive vision loss, like those with AMD, often begin to question their place in life and in the family, among other aspects of their identity. The view of the Bergman Institute is that without a reassessment of their own meaning and purpose, many people will have greater difficulty getting to a point of acceptance in their grieving process, which is necessary for moving forward in life. A particularly difficult aspect of vision loss for people of any age is adjusting to a life in which one may need to move from having as their ultimate purpose being the one who is there for others, without any perceived need for help from others, into becoming a person who requires assistance from family and friends.

The same person may also have found a lifetime of purpose and a great deal of meaning in being "the breadwinner" in the family but may suddenly face a change in this dynamic at the height of his or her earning years, depending on the age of disease onset. Redefining what it means to be a person with purpose thus requires much more time and a significantly greater effort for some than it does for others.

In dealing with this sometimes dramatic shift in one's identity, and in all other aspects of adjustment that vision loss can bring, the institute's licensed clinicians blend in their treatment approaches both cognitive-restructuring and psychodynamic techniques. The first is useful for identifying and neutralizing self-defeating and erroneous thoughts. Psychodynamic principles help patients work on relationship dynamics established earlier in life that can impact present well-being.

In addition to these techniques, we rely a great deal on the "existential" and "systems" schools of psychotherapy. We thus look at the person in the context of his or her own life goals and sense of purpose within his or her own life goals and social and familial surroundings. In fact, no empirically supported psychological approach is privileged over others in the clinic, which is part of what makes for an interesting and flexible treatment environment.

CONCLUSION

The establishment of a dedicated department, staffed in a multidisciplinary way and committed to both treatment and training is novel, both at The Lighthouse and in the vision rehabilitation field at large. This addition was central to the comprehensive model ushered in by the administration of the agency and the low vision clinic in recent years (see the Prologue to Part 2 of this book). And while many patients who come to The Lighthouse will never seek or need the services offered by the Bergman Institute, the staff is here for the many who accept the help offered, either after self-reflection on that need, or by the urging of those who know and love them.

NOTES

1. Amy Horowitz, Joann P. Reinhardt, and Kathrin Boerner, "The Effect of Rehabilitation on Depression among Visually Impaired Older Adults," *Aging & Mental Health* 9 (2005): 563–70; Amy Horowitz, Joann P. Reinhardt, and Gary J. Kennedy, "Major and Subthreshold Depression among Older Adults Seeking Vision Rehabilitation Services," *American Journal of Geriatric Psychiatry* 13, no. 3 (2005): 180–87.

2. American Psychiatric Association, *Diagnostic and Statistical Manual of Mental Disorders,* 4th ed., Text Revision (Washington, DC: The Association, 2000).

3. Cynthia Owsley, Gerald McGwin, Paul P. Lee, Nicole Wasserman, and Karen Searcey, "Characteristics of Low-Vision Rehabilitation Services in the United States," *Archives of Ophthalmology* 127, no. 5 (2009): 681–89.

4. Patricia Grant, William Seiple, and Janet Szlyk, "The Impact of Depression on the Actual and Perceived Effects of Reading Rehabilitation for People with Central Vision Loss," *Journal of Rehabilitation Research and Development* 48, no. 9 (2011).

5. Amy Horowitz, Robin Leonard, and Joann P. Reinhardt, "Measuring Psychosocial and Functional Outcomes of a Group Model of Vision Rehabilitation Services for Older Adults," *Journal of Visual Impairment & Blindness* 94, no. 5 (2000): 328–37.

6. Meri Vukicevic and Kerry Fitzmaurice, "Butterflies and Black Lacy Patterns: The Prevalence and Characteristics of Charles Bonnet Hallucinations in an Australian Population," *Clinical and Experimental Ophthalmology* 36 (2008): 659–65.

7. Robert Yacoub and Steven Ferrucci, "Charles Bonnet Syndrome," *Optometry* 82 (2011): 421– 27.

8. Geoffrey Schultz and Robert Meizack, "The Charles Bonnet Syndrome: 'Phantom Visual Images,'" *Perception* 20, no. 6 (1991): 809–25.

9. Vukicevic and Fitzmaurice, "Butterflies and Black Lacy Patterns."

10. It is important to emphasize that the well-known and sometimes controversial stage model published in the landmark book *On Death and Dying* (London: Routledge, 1969) was originally presented by Dr. Kübler-Ross in relation to the reactions of the *dying* *person* and not, as later popularized by advocates of the theory, in relation to the survivors' process of grieving the loss of a loved one—an application whose appropriateness is in far more doubt (see, for example, Ruth Davis Konigsberg, *The Truth about Grief: The Myth of Its Five Stages and the New Science of Loss* [New York: Simon & Schuster, 2011]).

An interesting footnote to this topic is that Dr. Kübler-Ross was working at The Chicago Lighthouse in the capacity of a psychiatrist, as well as at Chicago's Billings Hospital, during the time she was believed to have formulated this model.

CHAPTER 10

The Low Vision Eye Exam

What to Expect

Kara Crumbliss

Most individuals who have macular degeneration have experienced some loss of vision, known as *low vision*. Low vision refers to difficulty in seeing the things an individual wants to see, even while using the best spectacles or contact lenses available. Standard medicine or surgical interventions also will not restore reduced vision.

Although low vision cannot be corrected, people with low vision often benefit from low vision rehabilitation. *Low vision rehabilitation* is a specialty area of eye care that focuses on improving a person's visual function. In low vision rehabilitation, the focus is shifted from diagnosing and treating the eye disease to addressing the day-to-day difficulties caused by low vision and maximizing the remaining vision.

Common examples of activities that people with macular degeneration and subsequent low vision have difficulty with include reading, writing, recognizing faces, seeing in bright or dim lighting, and driving. A low vision examination focuses on such difficulties and works to find devices and other solutions that will allow individuals to perform these everyday activities with their low vision. In many instances, people with macular degeneration can regain some visual function by using prescribed low vision devices to assist them with reading, writing, seeing faces, continuing hobbies, and, occasionally, even driving. (Low vision devices make use of lenses or other technology to make visual information more viewable and to meet a person's visual goals.) This chapter discusses who might benefit from a low vision examination, where to find a low vision specialist, who is on the rehabilitation team, what a low vision exam entails, and some of the low vision devices that are available.

WHO BENEFITS FROM A LOW VISION EXAM?

The first step in knowing whether a low vision examination would be helpful to an individual is for that person to consider a few questions:

+ Do I have trouble seeing the things I want to see?
+ Have I stopped doing something because of my vision loss that I would like to resume?
+ Am I willing to try using a device to help me see, even if it looks different from a typical pair of eyeglasses?

If the answer to these questions is yes, then a low vision examination is likely to be both educational and helpful. After all, when people lose hearing, they generally obtain an evaluation and a hearing aid from an audiologist. They don't just stop listening, and they don't buy just any device from a corner store without consulting a specialist. An individual who loses vision owes him- or herself no less.

When devices such as magnifiers are purchased from unreliable sources such as magazines, the Internet, or a local store without proper guidance, these purchases are often poor investments, as they frequently are not effective for an individual's specific visual condition. Even if an individual has tried to use a magnifier unsuccessfully in the past, if he or she has not had a low vision exam and is still answering yes to the previous questions, a low vision exam may be helpful.

When an individual notices a loss of vision, he or she should first see an eye care specialist, either an ophthalmologist or an optometrist, to find out what is causing the problem. However, once macular degeneration is identified as the cause of the problem, additional care from a low vision specialist is crucial. A *low vision specialist* is a specially trained ophthalmologist or optometrist who conducts a special type of examination and prescribes specific low vision devices and services to improve the visual function of people who have low vision. The low vision examination measures an individual's remaining vision, and then low vision devices such as magnifiers, telescopes, lights, and filters, as appropriate, may be used to amplify images, similar to the way a hearing aid amplifies sound. In addition to optical and nonoptical devices, a range of services may be planned such as training in the use of devices, in orientation and mobility (O&M) techniques for independent movement, and in activities of daily living.

Anyone with macular degeneration ought to be monitored closely by an eye care specialist (ophthalmologist,

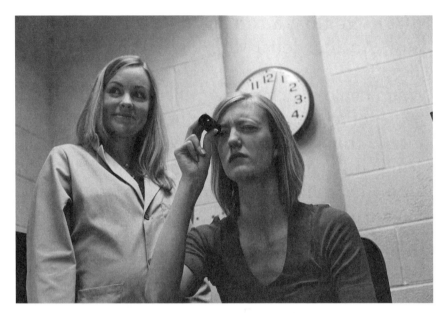

Dr. Crumbliss demonstrating the use of a telescope to a patient. (The Chicago Lighthouse for People Who Are Blind or Visually Impaired)

retinologist, or optometrist). Yet, despite monitoring and even some medical treatments, it is likely that such a patient will still not be able to perform many everyday tasks, since the damaged macula of the eye is responsible for the detailed central vision people require to perform many daily activities, such as reading; seeing street signs; recognizing faces; participating in visual hobbies such as bingo, card playing, and reading music; cooking; and even dialing the phone.

Losing the ability to do these tasks can be both overwhelming and frightening. It may even seem pointless to continue to undergo treatments for macular degeneration when the patient's vision does not improve. Each visit to the eye care specialist may serve as a reminder that a person still can't see what he or she wants to see. However, low vision devices and learning certain techniques for carrying out daily activities can help, and the low vision examination is the first step in obtaining those services.

WHO PROVIDES LOW VISION CARE?

Although there are many centers and clinics across the country that provide low vision services, the professionals who provide the services may vary. A low vision specialist may be either an optometrist or an ophthalmologist, who will work with the patient to assess his or her vision needs and design a rehabilitation plan of care. The low vision specialist may then involve other professional services in a plan for the patient, including counseling, rehabilitation therapy, orientation and mobility, technology, and vocational specialists as needed to ensure that comprehensive services are offered.

As discussed in Chapter 9, adjusting to vision loss can require time and professional guidance. *Social workers* or *psychologists* may meet with the patient to identify how he or she is adjusting to the vision loss and offer strategies for adjusting and accepting it. Support groups and individual counseling can be helpful in coming to terms with this loss.

Certified low vision therapists, vision rehabilitation therapists, or *occupational therapists* may provide training in the use of low vision devices recommended by the low vision specialist. Evaluation and training in the effective use of devices and strategies may be offered in an office or in the patient's home environment to ensure that the devices are meeting a person's needs and addressing his or her goals. The therapists may also teach methods of carrying out everyday activities with low vision and adapting the home environment with *nonoptical low vision devices* (items that promote independent performance of a task but do not involve optical lenses, such as lighting, large print, or auditory devices) to make it safer and easier to function. Some examples of nonoptical low vision devices are talking watches and clocks, big-button phones, and large-print checks.

Orientation and mobility instructors may work with an individual to evaluate his or her mobility skills and provide strategies on how to travel safely despite one's vision loss. *Technology consultants* may work with an individual to evaluate devices such as electronic magnifiers, computer adaptations such as large keyboards, and screen enlargement and reading systems. *Vocational counselors* work with individuals who have employment goals to help meet them. These goals may include finding employment, keeping employment, or acquiring education for eventual employment in a particular field.

These are just a few of the professionals that a person with vision loss might interact with during the rehabilitation process. Despite the wide variety of professionals involved in the process, the rehabilitation plan will be designed and overseen by the low vision specialist, who needs to coordinate the efforts of these professionals (possibly with the assistance of a case manager) to ensure that the patient will get all of the services he or she needs.

FINDING LOW VISION SERVICES

Often patients are not aware of the existence of low vision services or where to find them. A low vision rehabilitation examination and plan of care are different from a routine eye examination and the treatment for an eye disease. Both are very important. One should not replace the other, as they complement each other. An eye care specialist monitors eye diseases, watches for signs of progression, and offers treatment when available that may delay or slow the progression of vision loss from macular degeneration. A low vision specialist will work to maximize the remaining vision. Without care from both specialists, an individual with macular degeneration risks further vision loss or continued loss of visual function. In some instances, an eye care specialist who is knowledgeable about low vision may also provide low vision examinations and can serve both purposes.

Locating a specialist, practice, or clinic nearby that provides low vision examinations doesn't need to be difficult. The following are a few places for patients to begin:

✦ An individual can start by asking his or her eye care specialist about low vision services and for a recommendation of local specialists or practices.
✦ The American Optometric Association (www.aoa.org) has a section on its website listing vision rehabilitation professionals, as does the American Academy of Ophthalmology (www.aao.org). (See the Resources section for more information.) The websites of both organizations, and other Internet resources, can help in finding low vision specialists.
✦ Local and regional university teaching hospitals' eye care departments may offer low vision rehabilitation programs or supply recommendations.
✦ Friends or family members can assist an individual in looking on the Internet or in telephone directories if using these resources is difficult with his or her current vision.

Making the Appointment

It is important for prospective patients to call and speak with someone at the low vision clinic or practice about what their services entail and to discuss fees. The clinic or practice will also likely provide guidelines to help them prepare for an appointment. Although many insurance companies will cover the fees for a low vision examination, most do not cover the fees for *refraction* (the assessment of the prescription for ophthalmic lenses, including magnification lenses, to improve vision) or for low vision devices. The clinic may offer guidance on the expected costs and what health insurance is likely to cover. A patient can also speak with his or her insurance carrier prior to or after the examination about what may be reimbursed.

If finances threaten to prevent a patient from getting needed care and devices, he or she should inquire at the practice about available funding options. Some low vision clinics have grants and funding sources that they may be able to offer patients in order to pay for care or devices. The practice may be able to recommend lending institutions that can provide low-interest credit for purchase of low vision devices. Some local agencies and not-for-profit organizations such as Lions Clubs chapters may be able to offer assistance to patients in financial need. Finally, some state-funded rehabilitation programs may be offered through a state's department of rehabilitation services or department of human services. Contacting a state department or agency may help in finding resources in one's local area.

Preparing for the Appointment

The more prepared a patient is for the appointment, the better the time spent with the low vision specialist. It is important to bring the following items to the appointment:

+ Insurance cards and photo identification
+ A list of all medications and any health problems or previous surgeries. The specialist will want to know about

health issues, and it is easy to forget some of these items if they are not written down.

+ A copy of the report from the patient's most recent eye examination if available. This will help the specialist know about current and past treatments.

+ Any eyeglasses currently worn and also any eyeglasses that were prescribed but are no longer worn because the patient feels they no longer work.

+ Any magnifiers or other devices currently or previously used. The specialist will look at all of these to ensure that any new devices that are recommended are an improvement over what is being used currently or has been tried in the past.

+ A list of objects the patient struggles to see, along with some samples, such as books, magazines, or playing cards. The samples will allow the patient to try devices while in the eye care office to ensure they work on what he or she wants to see.

The patient will need to arrange transportation to the facility where the examination will take place. Many people with low vision don't drive, and asking a friend or family member to drive them may seem like an inconvenience. However, this person can also play a key role in the examination. Even if the patient can drive or travel alone by public transportation, it is recommended that he or she bring someone else to the examination who can serve as a "coach." The coach acts as a second set of ears, may take notes, and helps remember the important information discussed during the examination.

Most patients have a lot of questions they want to ask the specialist. Again, it is a good idea to write them down beforehand. "Sample Questions to Bring to the Low Vision

Sample Questions to Bring to the Low Vision Exam

1. Will my macular degeneration get a lot worse?
2. Can you give me better eyeglasses?
3. I want to read (books, newspapers, magazines, large-print books). Can you prescribe a device that will help me do this?
4. Is there a support group you can recommend?
5. Can I still drive?
6. I can't drive anymore. Can you suggest some transportation alternatives?
7. The sunlight bothers my eyes a lot. Why does this happen, and what can I do to prevent this?
8. What can I do or use to see the television screen better?
9. How can I improve my vision when looking at a computer screen?
10. I am having difficulty writing. What can I do that will help me?
11. I want to do crossword puzzles but cannot see the print. What can I use to help me see the page better?
12. Where can I get access to books or newspapers in audio formats?
13. Am I visually impaired or legally blind? Can you give me documentation of this?
14. Can you help me with resuming a former activity (such as sewing, crocheting, playing golf)?
15. My depth perception and balance seem off, and I am fearful of falling. What causes this, and what can be done to improve my safety?

Exam" is a list of some typical questions that patients often have.

THE LOW VISION EXAMINATION

This section describes the different steps in the low vision examination and how low vision rehabilitation differs from general eye care.

To put it simply, the low vision examination consists of three As:

✦ **Asking** about a patient's needs and goals.
✦ **Assessing** a patient's eyes and vision and helping him or her understand his or her eye condition and functional vision, that is, the way the patient is able to use his or her remaining vision in performing real-life tasks, not the way a person reads an eye chart in the office.
✦ **Adapting** tasks with devices to help meet the individual's needs and goals.

Overall, the purpose of the low vision examination and consultation is to improve the patient's functional vision, that is, how he or she uses vision to perform everyday activities.

The American Optometric Association low vision section and the American Academy of Ophthalmology publish established standards for performing low vision examinations. This consistency is intended to ensure that no matter which low vision specialist an individual goes to, the examination will tend to be the same or similar. The parts of the examination one can expect are case history, vision assessment, refraction, device assessment, ocular health assessment, and rehabilitation plan of care.

Case History

An essential part of a low vision examination is the case history, which is taken at the beginning of the examination. The low vision specialist or team members, such as social workers and psychologists, gather information, such as age, eye condition, and other health conditions of the patient. It is important for the specialist to be aware of any other health conditions, so that the entire health and well-being of the patient as they relate to the person's vision may be addressed. Some health conditions and medications have the potential to affect a person's visual system. A specialist will want to determine, for example, if a person with diabetes can see his or her blood sugar monitor and, if needed, is able to measure his or her insulin despite the vision loss. Or a person with arthritis may have difficulty holding a magnifier. Being aware of such health conditions will guide the specialist in prescribing the device that will work best for the patient.

The specialist will also ask about eye surgeries or injuries, including any cataract surgeries, that a person may have undergone, to determine the stability of the eye condition and any other eye conditions that may affect vision. For example, if a person's macular degeneration is actively exudative, or "wet," as described in Chapter 8, a patient may be receiving treatments that may make his or her vision unstable. In such instances, the specialist may need to postpone prescribing low vision devices or adjust the low vision prescriptions as treatment progresses. Still beginning low vision rehabilitation during this time is most often recommended.

The patient will also be asked about day-to-day activities and how his or her vision has affected them. Questions about support systems, such as family and friends, are important, since a person will need support in dealing with vision loss. A person's macular degeneration will also affect the lives of the people around him or her. Family members or friends often are encouraged to accompany the patient to the examination, so that they, too, can understand what the patient is coping with. Family members may not understand, for example, why a person can see some things and not others, such as when a person complains that he or she can't read but can clearly see a dropped coin on the floor. Being present at the examination will help family members better understand a patient's vision.

The specialist will also ask how a person functions under different visual conditions, such as in bright or dark environments, when seeing colors, in situations involving depth perception, and while traveling. All these activities may be affected by macular degeneration. Then the patient will work with the specialist to identify a list of specific visual goals. One example of a visual goal might be to obtain a device that will allow the patient to read the newspaper. Another might be to obtain a filter to control outdoor glare that is bothering him or her. Depending on the person's vision, all of these goals may not be realistic. The specialist and the patient will work together throughout the examination to achieve these goals and then modify those that aren't achievable until the person's vision has been maximized for as many tasks as possible. Once the patient and doctor have formulated this list of goals, the specialist will assess the patient's visual system using various tests and measures.

Vision Assessment

Vision assessment typically begins with a person being asked to read a distance eye chart. The eye chart used in low vision examinations usually differs from those used in regular eye examinations. Low vision charts are usually not projected on the wall as is typical at most routine eye examinations. Instead, the chart is usually on a stand, so that it can be moved to a distance at which it is visible to a patient; it may have larger letters and numbers, allowing the patient's vision to be measured accurately. Thus, a patient who is unable to see the letters on a regular eye chart may be surprised to discover that he or she can read the letters or numbers on the low vision chart because the letters on the chart are bigger and are positioned closer to the person. This experience may be the patient's first introduction to the concept and benefits of magnification: If something is larger, it's easier to see; if something is closer, it is easier to distinguish (a concept known as *relative distance magnification*).

The low vision specialist will also encourage the patient to move his or her eye off center and use peripheral vision to read the eye chart. This technique is called *eccentric viewing.* A person with macular degeneration may have already discovered that he or she can see things better if he or she doesn't look directly at them because central vision has been damaged by the disease. Looking off center allows the person to use undamaged peripheral or side vision to help him or her see and recognize objects. Together, the specialist and the patient work to identify the direction in which the patient should look to achieve the clearest image. This *eccentric viewing point* corresponds to an undamaged area of the retina closest to the macula (see Chapter 8) that an individual can use to see best; this point, once identified, is known as the *preferred retinal locus (loci)*. The specialist may be able to show the patient this point on his or her retina if there is a picture of the patient's retina available to view.

A specialist may also use other tools and methods to determine which part of the retina is healthy and which part is damaged. *Scanning laser ophthalmoscopy* and *microperimetry technology* are techniques in which instruments are used to identify and plot *scotomas* (missing areas of vision) in relation to functional areas of vision in a person's eye. They can also help with locating the preferred retinal locus. The specialist will work to reinforce the use of this area in eccentric viewing and may even give the patient homework to practice using this spot more efficiently when attempting to view an object.

Measurements of near vision (the vision used to look at objects approximately 16 inches or closer, as in tasks such as

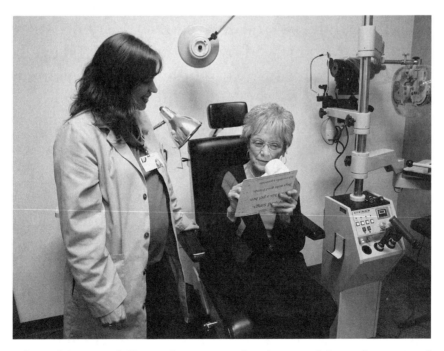

A low vision specialist evaluates a patient's near vision using a stand magnifier to read a test card. (The Chicago Lighthouse for People Who Are Blind or Visually Impaired)

reading) will be made using near vision charts. Measurements of intermediate vision (the vision used to view objects from approximately 16 to 30 inches away, such as a computer screen) may also be made, depending on the individual's goals. In addition, the specialist may, for example, use additional lighting and low-contrast charts to determine how a person might function visually in different situations. In regard to reading, black ink printed on white paper, as in a book, will typically provide more contrast than newspaper print on a grayish background. In general, people with macular degeneration have a more difficult time with low-contrast tasks, such as reading newspaper print, and an individual's performance in this area is important for a low vision specialist to note.

As part of the examination, a low vision specialist may repeat these measurements while the patient is wearing eyeglasses and using other devices, to determine the current effectiveness of the device for the patient. A patient should not be discouraged by how far down the eye chart he or she can or cannot read. These initial measurements help the specialist to determine the appropriate magnification power of the devices that may be prescribed. An individual who cannot read a particular line on an eye chart may simply need a higher-powered device to achieve his or her goals. Not being able to reach them initially does not necessarily mean that he or she cannot ultimately achieve them.

The low vision specialist may perform additional tests, including an examination of a patient's eyes, pupils, and eye movements, as well as a patient's color vision, before or after the next portion of the examination. Eye dominance—the preference for using one eye over the other—may also be tested. If an individual's poorer seeing eye is dominant, he or she might need to practice over time to learn to use the eye that has better vision—similar to the way a person accustomed to using the right hand to write would need to practice to learn to use the left hand. The eye care specialist may recommend using a patch over the dominant eye or some visual training exercises to improve the function of the nondominant eye.

Refraction

A refraction is usually the next step in the low vision exam. *Refraction* is the process by which a specialist observes how light passes through the patient's eye and is bent by the eye's lens and added external lenses to ensure it is in focus on the retina. Light must be focused at the retina in order for anyone to see as clearly as possible, regardless of whether an individual has macular degeneration or wears eyeglasses. By performing a refraction test, the specialist can determine the prescription for eyeglasses, if any, that will provide the patient with the clearest image, or whether any further improvement to the patient's current eyeglasses can be made. In some instances, wearing prescription eyeglasses may not help improve vision in patients who have retinal damage from macular degeneration.

Most people have had a refraction during their routine eye examinations. These refractions were likely done with the use of a *phoropter,* an instrument containing several lenses that eye specialists use to determine a patient's prescription. The patient looks through the phoropter during an eye examination while the specialist tries out different lenses and asks the patient to indicate which makes the object on a chart appear clearer.

A low vision refraction differs from a regular refraction in a number of ways. First, instead of a phoropter, a *trial frame* will likely be used. The trial frame is a device that looks like a pair of eyeglasses and is worn by the patient. The specialist inserts and removes lenses in the frame manually. The trial frame is useful because it allows the patient to use his or her peripheral vision, whereas a phoropter restricts a person's field of view to central vision and does not easily accommodate eccentric viewing. A trial frame is also most similar to how eyeglasses function. Using a trial frame when refracting someone with macular degeneration will ensure that the patient is allowed to make use of eccentric viewing and that the selected lens focuses the image on the preferred retinal locus.

Second, the trial frame refraction technique allows for lens choices that are within a person's just noticeable difference. *Just noticeable difference* (sometimes abbreviated JND) refers to the difference in lens powers that is large enough for a person to notice a difference and determine which lens is better despite his or her loss of vision. The phoropter provides lens changes in small increments that are indicated for someone with vision that is 20/50 or better. Many people with macular degeneration have visual acuity poorer than 20/50, and the trial frame allows for adjusting the lens choices to a person's specific JND.

Despite careful refraction, many people with macular degeneration may not benefit from new eyeglasses because refraction ensures only that light and images are focused on the retina. If no focusing problem exists, and the light that passes through a person's eye is already focused on the retina, refractive eyeglasses or a change in an existing prescription will not be helpful. In this case, the problem lies solely with the retinal degeneration. Focusing an image on the retina can be likened to focusing a camera that uses film. A camera's focus can be refined by adjusting the lens before a picture is taken, but if the photograph is blurry because the film in the camera is damaged, refocusing won't help. Similarly, if damage to the retina is the primary cause of impaired vision, refocusing the eye will not improve vision.

After investigating whether new eyeglasses will be helpful for the patient with macular degeneration, other magnifying optical devices are tried next.

Device Assessment

Once the specialist has ascertained that light passing through a patient's eye is focused on the retina, the person's best visual acuity is measured with any prescription lenses in place. This is known as *best corrected visual acuity.* As described in Chapter 7, if a person's best corrected visual acuity is 20/200 or worse or if his or her visual field at its widest diameter is no greater than 20 degrees, the person is considered legally blind in the United States. Patients may need to be reminded that legal blindness is a term used for certain classification purposes, such as determining eligibility for disability insurance, and does not mean that the person is going to lose all vision.

Knowing a person's visual acuity will help the low vision specialist determine what devices a patient will need to achieve his or her goals. Common optical formulas are used to determine the strength of the magnification a patient will need in a device. Often, the magnifiers a patient may have tried in the past may not have worked because they weren't strong enough. Most higher-strength magnifiers have to be prescribed by a specialist; those bought without a prescription are not likely to be as strong.

To understand why the stronger magnifiers work, consider the vision of someone who has been classified as legally blind with 20/200 vision.

As explained in Chapter 7, when an individual is said to have 20/20 vision, what he or she recognizes and identifies accurately at 20 feet is what an average sighted person also recognizes and identifies at 20 feet. A person with 20/200 vision recognizes and identifies accurately at 20 feet what an average sighted person recognizes and identifies at 200 feet. Essentially, if a person's vision is 20/200, he or she needs to be 10 times closer to an object than a person with "normal" vision to recognize the object, or the object needs to be made larger so he or she can recognize it. An object can effectively be made larger with optical devices such as magnifiers and telescopes, but they need to be of the appropriate strength for the individual's vision. The low vision specialist will show the patient a variety of these low vision devices, depending on the patient's goals.

Magnifiers

Magnifiers come in many forms; they can be mounted in eyeglasses (spectacle magnifiers or spectacle microscopes), held in one's hand (handheld magnifiers), or stand on their own (stand magnifiers). Magnifiers are most commonly prescribed for reading. A person who uses a spectacle magnifier will have to hold reading material closer than he or she is used to, possibly even as close as one to two inches away. Although this may be difficult to get used to, it can be done. The benefit is that hands are kept free for other tasks, such as hobbies like knitting, playing cards, playing an instrument, and woodworking. If performing these types of activities is on a person's list of goals, a specialist may recommend a spectacle-mounted magnifier.

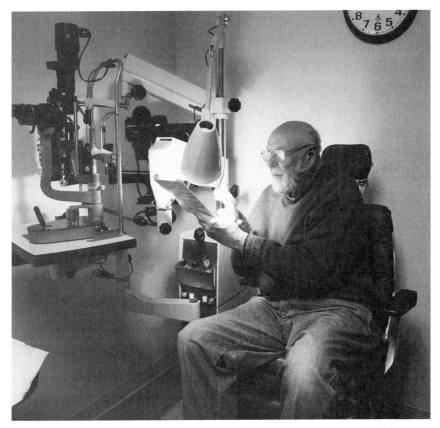

A patient tries using a handheld magnifier to read a book. (The Chicago Lighthouse for People Who Are Blind or Visually Impaired)

Handheld magnifiers are very useful, because they may offer a more comfortable viewing distance than lenses mounted in eyeglasses while still providing significant magnification. The disadvantage of using a handheld magnifier is that a person must be able to use a hand to hold the magnifier steady and maintain a certain distance from the item being viewed to keep the image in focus. For this reason, reading for long periods while using a handheld magnifier could become tiring.

Stand magnifiers can solve problems related to keeping the magnifier in focus because they stand independently. A person simply moves the magnifier over the reading material or other item and does not have to struggle to maintain the correct distance between the magnifier and text being read to maintain focus.

Both hand and stand magnifiers may require that the material be held along with the magnifier. This requires two working hands. If a person does not have the ability to use both hands, because of arthritis, for example, the doctor can consider a reading stand to be used with the magnifier. This adaptation holds the material for the user, so that only one hand is then necessary to manipulate the magnifier. A stand magnifier is often a better option in this case as it can stand on its own and be moved by pushing instead of grasping. In the case that function of both hands is compromised, such as arthritis in both hands, a stand magnifier and reading stand are a good option in optical magnifiers if spectacle magnifiers aren't well tolerated.

For both handheld and stand magnifiers, the field of view (or the area that can be seen at one time) decreases as the magnification power is increased, as a result of the optical laws of physics. For this reason, these magnifiers are not suited to viewing an entire page of print at once. A person whose goal is to read a larger portion of a page with a similar level of magnification will have to consider electronic magnifiers.

Electronic Magnifiers

Electronic magnifiers, also known as video magnifiers or closed-circuit television systems (CCTVs), are cameras equipped with software that enlarges the picture of an object or text projected onto a screen. They come in a variety of types, from desktop models to portable handheld devices. (These devices are discussed in more detail in Chapter 11.) Magnification in electronic magnifiers can

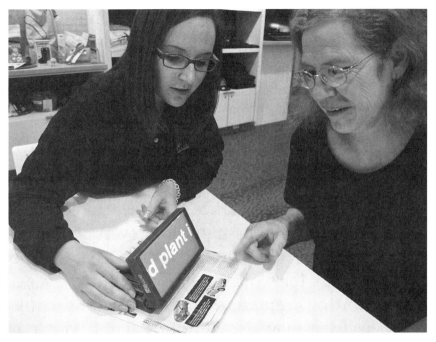

A staff member therapist demonstrates a portable electronic magnifier, showing how it can vary the color of the text displayed on the screen. (The Chicago Lighthouse for People Who Are Blind or Visually Impaired)

go as high as 60 times; traditional optical lens magnifiers typically don't exceed power higher than 15 times.

The low vision specialist may also consider electronic magnifiers for their other useful features. If a person's contrast sensitivity is reduced, the ability to distinguish objects that have lower contrast with their surroundings can be diminished. For example, newspaper print is lower contrast (grayer or dimmer) than black computer print on a bright white sheet of paper. A person with reduced contrast sensitivity would typically have difficulty seeing something like low-contrast newspaper print. Electronic magnifiers have the ability to change the colors of the objects being viewed in contrast to their background. Using an electronic magnifier, the image of newspaper print can be made a darker black and the background whiter, thereby increasing the contrast. The contrast can also be reversed on the electronic magnifier, to have white letters on a black background, which many people with macular degeneration find easier to see.

Telescopes

The low vision specialist may also look at ways to magnify objects viewed at a distance to make it easier for a person to see street signs, bus signs, and even people's faces. Telescopes and binoculars are two options that the specialist may consider. Telescopes are also useful for watching plays and sporting events and may be used for driving.

The specialist may also offer tips about how to make use of the principle that getting closer to objects has the effect of magnifying them, or *relative distance magnification,* to view objects usually viewed at a distance. For example, sitting closer to the television makes it easier to see what is on the screen, because the picture occupies a larger angle on the retina and stimulates both central vision and a larger area of peripheral vision. When an image occupies a larger area of the retina, it increases the chance that it will land on some of the undamaged peripheral areas outside the affected areas of the macula.

Devices for Driving

When meeting with a patient, the specialist should also discuss whether a person's current level of vision meets the requirements for driving in the state in which he or she resides. Each state is different, so it is important for the patient to ask the specialist about this requirement and to stop driving if his or her vision no longer meets it. Visual acuity, or one's ability to identify letters of a certain size on the eye chart, is only one aspect of the vision needed for driving, so the specialist may also want to perform additional tests, such as reaction time and peripheral visual field testing and awareness before discussing driving with the patient. In some states, if vision is reduced only slightly, to the point where a person needs a device to help see objects like street signs, the specialist may prescribe a special telescope to be worn while driving. This device, known as a *bioptic telescope,* may allow some individuals to continue driving legally despite some loss of vision.

Driving is a very complex task, and vision is only one component of it. Even if a specialist tells a patient that his or her vision still qualifies him or her to drive legally, if the person is not comfortable behind the wheel, he or she should consider this feeling a signal to stop driving. It is important for individuals to act responsibly and make this important decision for their own safety and the safety of others.

Filters and Lighting

Finally, the specialist will likely discuss sensitivity to light, or *photophobia*, and consider filters to help alleviate any sensitivity or glare a patient may be experiencing. Filters are similar to sunglasses but are different in that they are more selective in the wavelengths of light that they filter out. A person may have noticed that his or her vision is better when facing away from the sun, but seems much worse when facing it. Filters will filter out the wavelengths of light that are causing an individual to experience glare and allow the light needed to see well to pass through. The specialist will discuss which filters and lens treatment options might be most beneficial.

Other Equipment and Services

During the examination, the low vision specialist should also discuss other available tools, programs, and services. For example, Talking Books, auditory newspapers, support groups, operator-assisted dialing, and large-print resources, such as books, checks, and bill statements, are all available to assist a patient (some of which are described in detail in Chapter 4 in Part 1 of this book). (Many people don't know they can get large-print checks or request large-print bill statements.)

The specialist can explain how to obtain these services based on the patient's location or may refer the patient to a case manager or therapist to coordinate such services. The specialist should also discuss some of the other professional services mentioned earlier, such as counseling, orientation and mobility training, and working with a low vision therapist or occupational therapist to learn how to use low

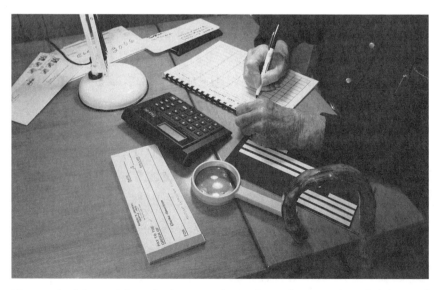

Nonoptical low vision devices, such as these large-print checks and check register, talking calculator, and envelope-addressing guide, promote independence in carrying out everyday tasks. (Earl Dotter/ American Foundation for the Blind)

vision devices and nonoptical aids, when formulating a plan of care.

Ocular Health Assessment

The low vision specialist will often want to look at a patient's retina and macula to be sure that the appearance of the patient's eye and retina correlates with the person's visual functioning. When vision loss doesn't correlate with the visible damage to the eye, the specialist needs to determine whether other eye problems may be compounding the problem. For example, if the vision of a person with macular degeneration is substantially reduced beyond what is typical with his or her degree of degeneration, and the patient also has a cataract, the cataract may be what is exacerbating the vision loss. Removing the cataract could provide some improvement to the vision.

In many cases, a person who is already under the care of a macular degeneration specialist may not need to undergo some of the assessment procedures outlined here. For example, the low vision specialist may defer to the macular degeneration specialist's findings and management and forego dilating a person's eye during an exam. Dilation is a procedure used to temporarily widen the pupil (the dark middle part of the eye that is surrounded by the colored portion of the eye known as the iris) using eye drops. This procedure is done when the physician needs a detailed view of all the structures lying at the back of the eye, including the macula and retina. A side effect of dilation is temporary blurring of vision. A low vision specialist, who is focusing on improving a person's functional vision, may avoid this procedure if the macular degeneration specialist has performed it recently and the records are available. If, for some reason, it is necessary to perform a dilation, it will be done at the end of the examination, so that the blurriness in vision doesn't interfere with the functional measurements reviewed earlier.

Rehabilitation Plan of Care

The low vision specialist will likely conclude the examination by recommending devices for the patient to try. Some other techniques to improve visual function may also be recommended. These might include using large-print checks, bold pens and bold-lined paper, large-print playing cards, audio books, talking watches, and so on. Many nonprescriptive adaptive devices such as these are available to help perform day-to-day activities.

The specialist will also typically make recommendations for the other professionals who may provide rehabilitation services to the patient. In some facilities, certified low vision therapists or occupational therapists will next work with the patient to train him or her in the use of the devices prescribed and to recommend nonoptical aids and services; in others, the specialist or other professionals may do this. Some low vision programs may also offer devices for loan, so that patients can try out different devices before making the decision to purchase one.

It is likely that an appointment will be made for the patient to come back for follow up to be conducted on how successful the patient has been in using the devices. The length of time between appointments will vary depending on the specialist. The specialist will also ensure that the patient continues to receive routine care and monitoring for macular degeneration by his or her regular eye care provider. This monitoring typically takes place at least every six months, and often sooner, depending on the severity of the patient's condition.

If a person is having trouble accepting his or her vision loss, the specialist may also recommend participation in local support groups or working with a counselor. Losing one's vision may feel like losing a family member, and grieving and time are necessary to help a person to adjust. As discussed in Chapter 9, needing time to deal with one's vision loss is normal and common, and counseling can help to overcome sadness and other emotions associated with the loss.

If a person has indicated that traveling independently is difficult or frightening, the specialist may recommend considering use of a white cane and making an appointment with an orientation and mobility (O&M) instructor. An O&M instructor will provide instruction in certain traveling techniques and tips on relying less on one's vision and more on one's awareness and other senses combined when traveling. An O&M instructor will also teach a person how to use a white cane safely and appropriately. White canes are also an important tool to let other people know that a person is visually impaired. They can assist when traveling, but one must be trained to use them; an O&M instructor is the person to help with this.

Finally, the examination should conclude with the specialist's reviewing a person's goals and the tools prescribed to achieve them. Depending on the severity of the vision loss, a letter from the specialist documenting a person's visual impairment or legal blindness might be provided to the patient, which will make him or her eligible for additional services, such as "411 free," or operator-assisted dialing, which will allow the person to call the operator and be connected to numbers without charge when reading the telephone book or dialing the phone is not possible.

AFTER THE EXAM

The duration of a low vision examination as described in this chapter may average between one and two hours. Once the low vision examination is over, it is time for the patient to go home and become an expert at using the low vision devices that have been prescribed for him or her, as discussed further in Chapter 11. An individual may find that a magnifier prescribed for reading books is also useful for reading labels on medicine bottles. A telescope prescribed for seeing faces can also be used to go bird watching. Each person must become the expert at choosing what device works best for him or her on each task. An individual may use a magnifier for a task that another person with macular degeneration may use for another task. A patient's personal preference will influence his or her choice. For example, one person may use his or her magnifier to read the mail and a spectacle magnifier to view and adjust the thermostat, while someone else may use a magnifier to view and adjust the thermostat and use his or her spectacle magnifier to read through the mail. Each individual must select the tool that best suits him or her for each task, as long as the tool gets the job done. There is no one right tool for everyone.

By the time of the next low vision examination, a person may be able to tell the specialist what works and what doesn't, and what goals still remain to be achieved. Patients need to remember that not every goal will be achievable, but many will be. If a person is frustrated about using a low vision device, he or she should see the low vision specialist to evaluate other devices. Patients need to keep in mind that using a device is a new way of seeing and that learning this process will take time, but eventually their skill will improve. It is also important to make sure they know that using their vision is to their benefit and will not worsen, exacerbate, or accelerate the disease of macular degeneration. Focusing on positive improvements and what can now be done again is helpful, rather than dwelling on what someone still can't do. With that positive mindset, patients with macular degeneration will find that vision rehabilitation services can offer both hope and improvements in everyday life.

CHAPTER 11

Integrating Low Vision Rehabilitation and Assistive Technology

Thomas B. Perski

For people who have macular degeneration or other eye diseases such as diabetic retinopathy or glaucoma, low vision rehabilitation services are available to assist with functional vision tasks. *Functional vision* refers to vision as it is used for everyday activities, rather than how it is measured in the eye care specialist's office.

As discussed in Chapter 10, low vision rehabilitation involves helping people with vision loss learn adaptive techniques, including the use of special technology known as low vision devices, to use their remaining vision to carry out everyday activities. The purpose of this process is to help people optimize their vision and continue to live an independent, satisfying life. Low vision services are typically aimed at people who have reduced vision in both eyes and need help with daily activities, which include but are not limited to such tasks as reading small print, writing letters or checks or filling out forms, cooking, sewing, seeing faces of grandchildren, and, for some people who need help with distance vision, reading street signs or even driving.

THE REHABILITATION PROCESS

Various professionals are involved in helping a person through the rehabilitation process, including optometrists, occupational therapists, low vision therapists, vision rehabilitation therapists, psychologists, and social workers. Professionals trained in assistive technology (also known as adaptive technology) play a role in visual rehabilitation by evaluating and training persons to use optical low vision and high-tech devices intended to help each person maximize his or her vision and to carry out tasks and activities that have been identified by the person as most important.

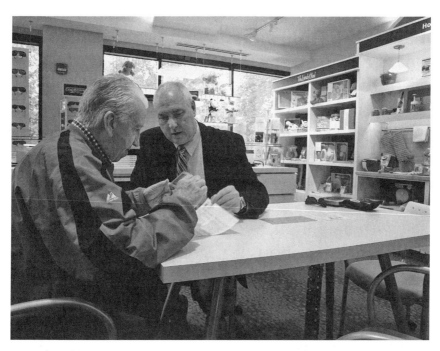

Mr. Perski demonstrates a portable video magnifier to a patient. (The Chicago Lighthouse for People Who Are Blind or Visually Impaired)

For the person receiving these services, it is helpful to consider each component of service as a learning process, that is, as an ongoing effort between patient and low vision professionals to constantly seek out new devices that will maximize available vision and to provide training in their use. In other words, it should not be expected that all will be cured with one appointment, that a single device will suffice for all types of tasks, or that the same device will continue to be the best solution for years on end. Instead, depending on the severity of the vision loss, low vision rehabilitation may be a process of different durations for different persons. For some, this process may need to be slow at first. Several aspects of the process may be going on simultaneously. Each part will take its time and must be completed in its entirety. Jumping from an early stage to a final solution is not recommended and will not result in successful outcome for most individuals. An essential part of the low vision professional's role, therefore, is educating patients about the nature of the process itself.

In general, patients should expect their low vision rehabilitation to be a slowly improving and constantly continuing course of action. However, there will be benchmarks throughout that will yield good solutions and improvements. If vision loss remains static, a person may remain pleased with a solution, and the rehabilitation process may pause for some duration. If vision worsens and the situation changes, however, the process will resume as the person will need to adapt and continue to seek out further solutions. This interplay between change and adaptation will continue for the rest of a person's life. Fortunately, this strategy should result in continued improvement and higher quality of life.

There are many low vision technology devices to help with a wide range of tasks performed by the person who experiences vision loss. These assistive technology devices provide a variety of different types of support and are increasing in number and variety each year. It is now almost always possible to access any type of print material, for example, regardless of the level of one's vision. In addition, tasks such as reading the mail and writing checks can be accomplished independently. For those who wish to access a computer or a cell phone or smart phone, the solutions are now available.

WHERE TO START

Historically, people sought assistance from a low vision center when their vision reached the 20/200 level, the point of legal blindness (see Chapter 7 for an explanation). Today, most specialists realize that it is far better to refer somebody for low vision services when they have mild to moderate vision loss in each eye, when solutions may be relatively simple. For instance, if a person's better-seeing eye is in the range of 20/50, and he or she is beginning to have trouble reading small print, sometimes a good reading or task light, with a stronger bifocal lens, can do the trick. Also, a small telescope, mounted in a pair of eyeglasses, might enable such a patient to see street signs or distant objects easily. In addition, there are special telescope eyeglasses for intermediate tasks, such as playing the piano or playing cards, that can help the person attain the equivalent of 20/20 vision.

Starting rehabilitation early on allows an individual to achieve a familiarity with using low vision devices and with making ongoing modifications in his or her use of them before his or her vision further deteriorates, a time when the person's patience may be thin and his or her attitude accordingly more negative. Once someone develops a fluency in using low vision tools, if his or her vision changes after the initial prescription and training, he or she may simply need to return to the low vision specialist for a quick "booster" session and to become skilled with the new device.

The Team Approach in Low Vision

Finding a low vision center that uses a team approach is typically best for the patient. In addition, working with a low vision optometrist, occupational therapist, or vision rehabilitation therapist who is trained and specializes in low vision before severe vision loss occurs is extremely important. It is also important to realize that low vision services are not medical services and do not treat the patient's eye condition; rather, they encompass rehabilitation with the goals of the patient's being able to perform everyday tasks and of improving the patient's quality of life. It is still essential for visits to the medical eye care specialist to be continued, but much benefit will come from also working with a low vision specialist for improvements in functional vision, or vision used to carry out necessary tasks.

The Role of the Patient

Unlike medical eye examinations, in which an eye care specialist may conclude with a diagnosis in a short amount of time, the entire low vision process can take many hours of direction and hard work. Individuals must stay focused, patient, and determined, not only during the examination, but in training themselves in properly using various devices, both optical and technological devices. Successful use of each device will be achieved through practicing many times a day, often for weeks. For example, using a closed-circuit television system (CCTV) or video magnifier requires daily practice for best results. Even an electronic Talking Book player can be confusing unless it is used daily until mastered. With guidance, training, and follow-up from vision rehabilitation professionals, best outcomes can be achieved by the patient with minimal frustration, confusion, and backtracking.

The patient needs to take ownership in this process; that is, to accept the responsibility that his or her commitment, dedication, and actions will in major part determine the success or failure of the overall procedure. Professional training, follow-up, and support are also critical. The low vision specialist may prescribe several devices for a patient. It is then the job of the patient to make progress in using those devices and work with the specialist and the low vision therapist to seek best solutions for any current and future situations. Simply put, it is unrealistic for the patient to expect that low vision professionals will automatically fix everything. It takes a lot of determined effort and strong will on the part of the patient to improve his or her life by trying to make the prescribed tools work.

A Variety of Tools

A common misconception about low vision devices is that there is one pair of eyeglasses or one technology device that will resolve everything. Actually, a typical low vision patient may use five or six different items on a daily basis to help with his or her visual tasks. Each device has a specific function, and the selection of an appropriate device relies heavily on whether, for example, one is reading small print or large print, reading at home versus reading a price tag in a store or a menu in a dark restaurant, or even trying to view the face of a grandchild or friend. There will not be one all-powerful item that will yield success in every situation; many tools will often need to be utilized.

Fortunately, a variety of products are widely available now. Devices ranging from the simplest handheld magnifier to high-tech items such as video magnifiers, computers, and headborn electronic goggles ensure that today's low vision patient may be independent and successful in whatever he or she wishes to accomplish—if he or she is willing to learn to do tasks in a different way, overcome some initial frustration, and find and sustain the patience to learn. Although it may take months of practice along with follow-up training before a person can perform tasks quickly and easily, the results are often well worth the effort.

LOW VISION TECHNOLOGY

At The Chicago Lighthouse for People Who Are Blind or Visually Impaired, there is a unique approach to all types of low vision and blindness technology, which is incorporated into almost every service provided by the agency. Integrated into the Low Vision Rehabilitation Service at The Chicago Lighthouse is a complete technology resource center where all persons are introduced to low vision technology after receiving their prescribed optical devices. These technology solutions may be software enlargement for the computer, a Talking Book player, a scanner that reads print aloud, or a video magnifier. A person may be referred to the technology department from the low vision optometrist, from the employment center, from the occupational therapist, or from psychological services, which employs a psychologist and a rehabilitation counselor (see Chapter 9). This integrated team approach encompassing many professional disciplines coupled with professional guidance is intended to give people the maximum opportunity to succeed with whatever technology they end up using, and, in turn, help them improve their quality of life.

Categories of Low Vision Technology

Access to Printed Material

Devices that facilitate access to printed material are the first main category of low vision technology. Historically, the *closed-circuit television reading machine* (CCTV), now commonly referred to as a *video magnifier,* has been the most popular low vision device worldwide.

Introduced in the mid-1970s, CCTV reading machines can display print material through a camera system with magnification beyond the capabilities of an optical device like a hand magnifier. For instance, a patient can turn the dial to display words from 3 times to 60 times the normal size. (These specifications are usually represented as 3X to 60X.) Also, the image can be manipulated to improve contrast. This is done through changing the colors of the letters and the background upon which they appear. For instance, white letters can be read on a black background or vice versa, or yellow letters on a blue background. The devices come with a variety of color combinations and can automatically switch the colors of the text one is reading to improve contrast between the letters and background and therefore increase the ease of seeing the print. Video magnifiers are low vision technology that allow people access to printed material and enable them to write as well.

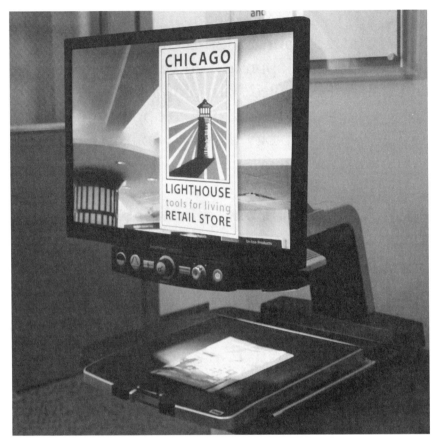

A closed-circuit television reading machine (CCTV), now commonly referred to as a video magnifier, can magnify text from 3 times to 60 times the normal size. (Eric Cromey)

Different types of video magnifiers are described in more detail later in this chapter.

Access to Computers

The second main category of low vision technology involves a person's access to computers. There are computer software programs known as *screen readers* that enable text to be read aloud through the use of *synthetic speech* (sometimes known as *text to speech*), which not only announces what is in a document but also reads the drop-down menu options and commands displayed on the computer's screen. These programs allow easy navigation around the many programs on the computer as well as the Internet. They will read aloud pretty much anything at which the computer's mouse points, such as the address bar, the tool bar, and drop down menus, and will also provide guidance to the user. Many users learn to navigate using keyboard commands rather than the computer mouse, eliminating the need to use vision.

In addition, there are voice recognition programs that allow a person to dictate text and have a computer type the words into a document. This *speech-to-text* software has come a long way and now recognizes words without the prior need for training the program to identify a person's unique voice. This type of program eliminates the need for a patient with low vision to rely heavily on the keyboard. Everything spoken into the microphone is displayed on the screen, and a process that makes writing a letter, e-mail, or essays much simpler.

Another kind of software is *screen magnification programs,* which enlarge the image on the computer screen. The effect is similar to that of a CCTV or video magnifier; the letters can be magnified from 1.5 times to 16 times the actual size. As with video magnifiers, the higher the magnification, the bigger the letters, but the smaller the portion of the page appearing on the screen. When using this type of assistive technology with a computer, the user needs to learn how to move the mouse back and forth to access the screen. There are many tips and tricks to learn, such as when to use magnification and when not to, what type of magnification works best for each person, and when the screen reader can be used in conjunction with magnification.

Getting the Most from Technology

The types of technology just described are amazing tools in providing access to the printed and electronic word. Through their existence and utilization, people with low vision have the same abilities as their fully sighted counterparts. However, technology is not a miracle cure. Learning to use these high-tech options has the same prerequisites as learning to use optical low vision devices. That is, people need to adopt a realistic perspective on and expectations of these tools and apply themselves to periods of sometimes difficult work to learn to use new devices and perform activities in a different way.

Learning the functions of each dial or button of a specific video magnifier, for example, as well as learning to view eccentrically (as described in Chapter 10), is key to success in using these devices. If a person has not read for some time, a schedule to help build up longer and longer reading times can be recommended. Learning to read on a video magnifier can often be slow and tedious, at first. Again, there is no easy fix. But although the process can be difficult, for many who are motivated the challenges will be overcome with persistence, and they will learn to use the video magnifier with speed and efficiency and accomplish many of their goals. At The Lighthouse hundreds of people have excelled at using a video magnifier or a computer far beyond what they originally thought they would be able to attain.

There are some realities that govern the use of every technological device about which users must know and be educated. Without this knowledge and understanding, a person will not approach each device with appropriate expectations of what the tool can accomplish. For most devices, reality may involve both positive gains and improvements along with negative side effects and limitations. For instance, as noted earlier, when text is enlarged on a video magnifier, the larger the magnification, the smaller the viewing area. Many users of video magnifiers would like to be able to see the whole page of a book or magazine at once, but most of the time, this is not possible, especially if the image on the monitor is magnified to such a degree that only a few words, or even one word, may be seen on the screen at a time. The more an image is enlarged, the more area on the screen will be consumed by fewer words, which appear much larger.

There is a solution to the inability to see more than a fraction of a page at one time, however. It is handled by a feature on traditional desktop video magnifiers known as

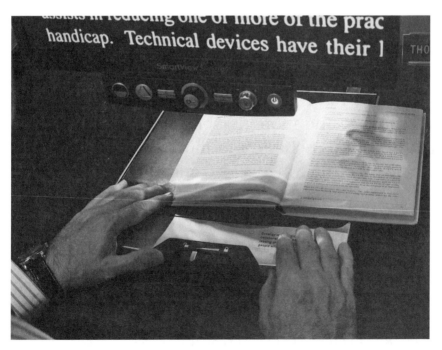

The X-Y table slides easily, moving the reading material resting on it and enabling the reader to scroll through the text on the screen. (Eric Cromey)

the X-Y table, which allows the person to scroll the text across the screen. The X-Y table is a flat surface on which the reading material sits below the camera of the device. It slides easily from side to side and from top to bottom, moving the reading material along with it. The view on the screen changes as the X-Y table moves. This situation is a perfect example of how the limitations of technology may be overcome. The X-Y table is a very beneficial aspect of the overall device, yet a difficult technique to utilize at first.

Smaller Lightweight Video Magnifier Technology

There are now a myriad of video magnifiers that are smaller and more lightweight than the traditional desktop models. Many of them couple to a person's own television or computer screen.

Arm-Mounted Video Magnifiers

One such device consists of a camera mounted on an arm. Some of these arms may be short, so that the camera is suspended 10 or 12 inches above the table. Other arms may be longer and more flexible, and the camera may be adjusted from 6 inches up to more than 24 inches above the table. Arm-mounted video magnifiers not only magnify writing and reading materials but also work well for persons who want to use them for crafts or hobbies. They usually cost less than other models, because these devices can be connected to existing televisions and computer screens, so it is not necessary to purchase a monitor. They usually do not come with an X-Y table, although many companies provide additional small, portable X-Y tables that can be purchased at any time.

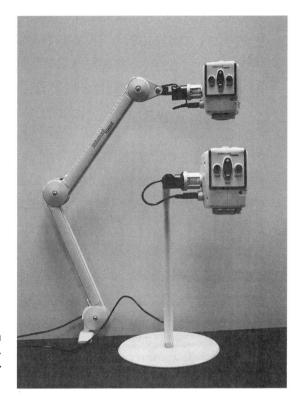

Arm-mounted video magnifiers can magnify writing and reading materials and work well for crafts or hobbies. (Eric Cromey)

Mouse Camera Video Magnifiers

Another category of video magnifier is a portable device sometimes known as a *mouse camera* because the camera is mounted in a small, handheld device that resembles a computer mouse. There are a variety of mouse-type cameras that work with both a standard television or a computer screen. There is even a mouse camera that connects to a laptop computer. Instead of moving an X-Y table, the person chooses the level of magnification he or she needs and then slowly moves the mouse across the print to read. These cameras are much less expensive than a desktop video magnifier, but they have some drawbacks. For instance, the range of magnification may be from only 7 to 20 times the original size.

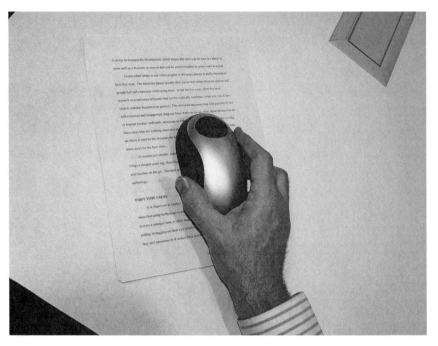

In a mouse camera video magnifier, the camera is mounted in a small, handheld device, and the image can be projected on a standard TV or computer screen. (Eric Cromey)

Portable Handheld Video Magnifiers

Portable handheld video magnifiers now exist that can be taken to a store to see food labels or used in a restaurant to read the menu. These items are usually battery-operated, and charging the batteries each night allows several hours of reading small print. This technology also has the capability of enlarging the text to many different sizes as well as improving the image through color and contrast options such as displaying white letters on a black background or colored letters on a white background.

OCR Scanning Systems

Another high-tech way to access print material is through the use of small, portable devices or desktop scan-

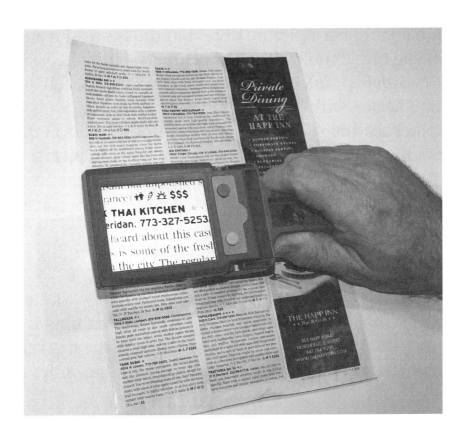

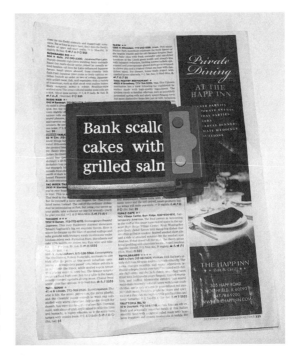

Portable handheld video magnifiers can be used to read print on the go. Color and contrast options include white letters on a black background. (Eric Cromey)

ners that can take a picture of text and then read it aloud. This type of technology, called *optical character recognition (OCR) scanning* and combined with text-to-speech technology, began with large, computer-based programs and computer scanners. Using these machines, a person could place a book on the scanner, close the lid, and push a button to let the computer access the image and then read it aloud. In the past, these devices were too expensive for many consumers to purchase. Also, some of these devices had to remain plugged into a power source, preventing their use with any type of mobility.

With advancements in today's technology, these devices are no longer large, can be easily used at home, and are now among the most portable tools on the market. In addition, they are more affordable. In contrast to yesterday's

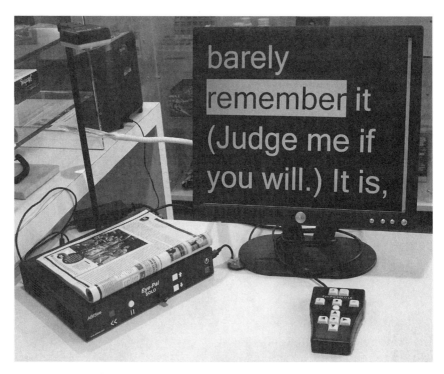

An OCR scanning system. (Eric Cromey)

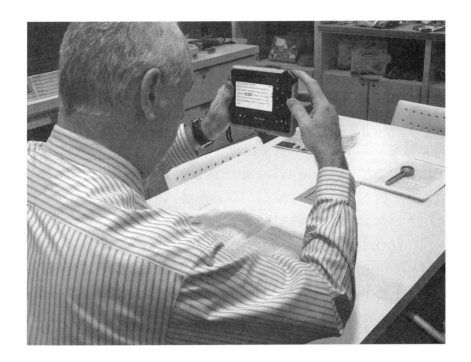

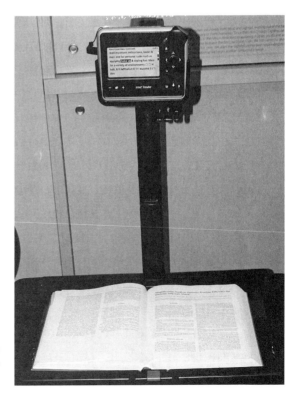

Some portable scanning devices can be handheld or set on a stand for hands-free viewing. (Eric Cromey)

large computer-based scanners that had to be plugged in, today's highly mobile devices can be held above a paper or book, take a picture of the page, and read the page's contents out loud anywhere. One such device utilizes a cell phone (more specifically the phone's camera and flash) to take the picture. With built-in special software and programming for people who are blind or visually impaired, this phone can be used to read virtually anywhere. Another similar device is about the size of a paperback book. It, too, has a camera and is held above a page to capture an image of the text, convert it to digital text, and then read it back to the user while displaying the words being read on its screen.

Video Goggles

Finally, there is a type of video magnifier that can be worn like a pair of goggles or binoculars. These battery-operated *video goggles* can help with seeing at a distance, such as viewing a concert or play, viewing items in a glass case at a museum or paintings at an art exhibit, and similar activities. Although these devices also have limitations in their field of view, they can magnify faces, so that a person could watch his or her grandchildren play on the floor or see the face of someone leading a religious service. These devices also have the ability to effectively increase or decrease illumination, which means that they can be used to see items in a dimly lit room such as a museum or concert hall as well as in brightly lit spaces such as a park.

People often refuse to use video goggles or telescopic spectacles in public, because of their appearance. Telescope lenses usually stick out several inches from the eyeglasses on which they are mounted, and people feel self-conscious when using them. Another reason these devices are less popular is that, ordinarily, telescope or video goggles cannot be used while moving. Most users who are walking must stop to view signs or other distant objects. Each time an object is seen in the distance, the telescope must be refocused by hand (similar to focusing binoculars) to obtain the best view. In the last few years, there has been research on a miniature telescope that can be surgically implanted inside one eye of a patient with age-related macular degeneration. If this device is approved for use in the general population, such a miniature telescope might help patients be less self-conscious and help them see faces while on the go.

The market for people who are blind or visually impaired is starting to see a trend in which one device is capable of being used in several different ways and serves a variety of unique purposes. An example is a cell phone with all of the usual features, such as calling capabilities, a calendar with a datebook, a contacts list, text messaging options, and so forth, which also reads the menus and commands aloud, can take pictures of text and read it aloud, and can be coupled with a talking GPS (global positioning satellite) program. Such high-tech tools are becoming more popular and enable the user with the power of multitasking. As screens get smaller, batteries become longer lasting, and more competition brings a cheaper price tag, these high-tech devices will become sleeker, more attractive, and function on the go. The next several years are likely to bring the development of more types of technology.

FIRST-TIME USERS

It is important to explain to patients some of the experiences that many individuals have when first using technology to assist with low vision. Many people state that when they first try a stronger lens, a video magnifier, or a magnified computer program, they feel a pulling or tugging on the eye that is uncomfortable and unfamiliar. Others state that they feel nauseous or that it makes their stomachs queasy, because of the strength of the lens or magnification and their closeness to the screen. These common reactions can be slowly overcome. As previously noted, low vision rehabilitation is often a time-consuming and sometimes difficult process of adjustment and cannot be hurried along, but steps toward becoming a successful user of a low vision device come with patience and forbearance.

Practicing reading in short spurts several times a day, every day, is the key. Patients should not overexert themselves, but rather, slowly, without skipping a single day, push themselves to do better over weeks and months. Professional training and follow-up are crucial to the patient's success. Some sales outlets for low vision technology do not provide proper training, so it is always best to find a low vision technology center that can provide this specific training.

THE FUTURE OF LOW VISION TECHNOLOGY

The future of low vision devices and assistive technology continues to expand and grow quickly. Some of the trends are easy to notice: the devices are getting smaller and more portable and seem to reflect the needs of our more mobile, on-the-go society. More and more companies are entering the marketplace with creative ideas as well. This competition is good for consumers, as it seems to be driving down prices and creating more innovation.

Another trend is the development of mainstream "off-the-shelf" consumer products with built-in accessibility. Smartphones with the capability of displaying large print or magnified print of many sizes, as well as audio and voice prompt menus, are already in the marketplace. Also, new applications are being developed for smartphone users to do such tasks as identify money, read the labels of food or drink packages, or read text from a page. The expansion of these new applications seems limitless and also helps innovation come to the marketplace at lower and lower costs. With time, more of these types of accommodations are likely to become more commonplace.

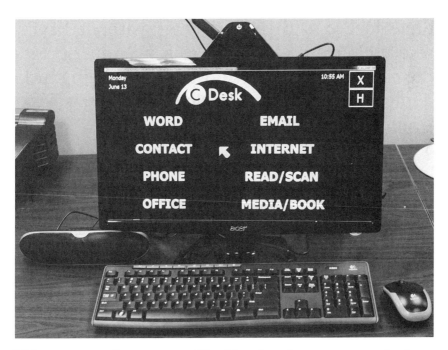

This program allows users with vision loss to use a computer for a variety of functions without advanced training in assistive technology. (Eric Cromey)

Imagine, for example, touch screen technology being used not only in conjunction with a computer, but also with a video magnifier reading machine! In this instance, the user will touch the word where he or she wants to begin reading, pinch the words directly on the screen to make them smaller, or release the pinch to expand the size of the letters on the screen.

Just recently, a new easy-to-use computer program called CDesk began offering a solution for both low vision and blind users, older people, or anyone who wishes to send e-mail, surf the Internet, scan and read books, listen to Internet radio, and download Talking Books, all on one program. This program will allow blind or low vision users a way to begin using a computer with only a few hours of training. There are also built-in capabilities to use voice commands and dictate letters and e-mails easily. CDesk will also allow those in the midst of vision loss to continue to access their computers without having to learn to use screen reader or screen magnifier programs. All these and many more innovations are being incorporated into new technology to help those with low vision to truly function like pros!

CHAPTER 12

The Impact of Macular Degeneration: An Epilogue

Patricia Grant

As discussed in Parts I and II of this book, age-related vision loss, specifically age-related macular degeneration (AMD), is one of the most common causes of visual impairment and blindness in the United States.[1] People who experience vision loss late in life typically do not undergo just the loss of visual function; they may also undergo a loss of independence, their social networks, and often the ability to enjoy life as they once did. More than a decade of research has demonstrated that a visual impairment is often accompanied by psychosocial reactions such as depression, anxiety, and emotional distress.[2]

PSYCHOSOCIAL FACTORS RELATED TO VISION LOSS

Depression

Past research has demonstrated a strong association between depression and age-related vision loss,[3] as well as a significant relationship between depression and declining visual functioning.[4] Depression has been found to be directly related to a decline in the ability to perform daily activities, independent of vision, age, and gender,[5] and is a more significant predictor for functional impairment than the severity of vision loss.[6] Older adults who are visually impaired report higher levels of depressive symptoms than older adults who are not visually impaired.[7]

Although there are a variety of low vision services available that serve to optimize remaining vision and thus improve quality of life, psychosocial issues are often neglected in the development of an overall treatment plan. Owsley et al.[8] reported that of all patients seen in vision rehabilitation centers in the United States, nearly half have problems with emotional or psychological adjustment, but only 11.8 percent of out-patient rehabilitation centers have a psychologist on staff. One reason for the lack of focus on psychosocial issues is the need for further investigation of how individuals with low vision are affected by depression and the benefits of addressing psychosocial issues within the treatment plans. With an understanding of the predictors of depression, more effective interventions can be developed that take these factors into account.

Although the link between depression and vision loss has been well established, what remains unclear is how depression may affect an individual in regard to visual function, adaptation to vision loss, and the success of treatment plans. A recent study investigating the relationship between depression and vision rehabilitation outcomes reported that those with greater depressive symptoms at the start of vision rehabilitation did not respond as well functionally to the goals of rehabilitation as those who did not report depression.[9] Yet, receipt of rehabilitative services are associated with trends toward lower levels of depressive symptoms, as counseling services, low vision clinical services, and use of adaptive devices have been shown to contribute to a significant reduction in depressive symptoms over time.[10] This finding suggests that the right combination of vision rehabilitative services can serve to increase use of functional vision and reduce depressive symptoms.[11]

Emotional Distress

Visual impairment that begins later in life can induce feelings of distress as an individual adapts to his or her vision loss. Emotional distress, in particular vision-specific distress, has been found to be the strongest predictor of depression.[12] Past research has suggested that such feelings are responsible for reductions in quality of life, as the individual experiences difficulty in carrying out daily activities.[13] Distress may also affect the way one may respond to the treatment of disease, as well as one's ability to manage the situation, as the greater the perception of risk of vision loss, the greater the feelings of distress may be, regardless of actual impairment.[14] One study reported that those who were legally blind in one eye were more distressed than those who were legally blind in both eyes, because they felt more at risk of losing vision in the other eye than those who already had experienced the full loss of vision. In addition, these authors found that when faced with vision loss, one's level of emotional stress affects the way one may cope with the disease and the ability to manage the situation.[15]

Coping and Adjustment

The ability to cope with vision loss may serve to reduce levels of emotional distress. Advancements have been made toward the understanding of how vision rehabilitation services may relate to coping strategies and specifically

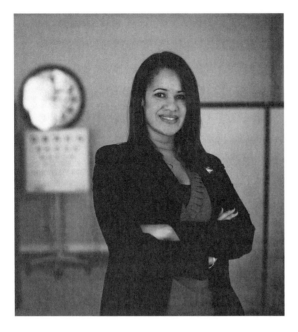

Patricia Grant in the Low Vision Research Laboratory. (The Chicago Lighthouse for People Who Are Blind or Visually Impaired)

to adaptation,[16] but further exploration needs to occur with regard to the most efficient types of coping patterns and how these strategies may predict better adaptation and serve to reduce distress, anxiety, and depression.

In general, the main focus of vision rehabilitation programs is to increase the level of the patient's functional ability with an overarching goal of helping people to adjust to life with a chronic disability. Vision rehabilitation may affect coping patterns of persons with a visual impairment either by promoting coping strategies or by raising awareness of the vision loss, which compels an individual to develop a coping strategy, or possibly both. Past research on coping with regard to adaptation has shown that use of active problem-focused coping rather than emotion-focused coping has led to better adjustment.[17] These outcomes also show that instrumental support, which consists of assistance from another, can be effective on a long-term basis, and suggest that vision rehabilitation can influence successful coping strategies and lead to better adaption over-all. This is an important concept, as many eye diseases are progressive and coping with the vision loss requires constant attention.

Social Support

The ongoing process of adaptation to visual impairment raises important challenges for relationships with friends and family members. Researchers have discussed the importance of social support systems when assessing quality of life and psychosocial well-being in patients with low vision. Social support has been found to be a critical factor in adaptation to stress in older adults[18] as well as a central contributor to the psychosocial well-being of patients with low vision.[19]

Instrumental support can be achieved through vision rehabilitation and can lead to better adaptation. Higher levels of life satisfaction, lower levels of depressive symptomatology, and better adaptation to vision loss have been found to be associated with greater perceived emotional support from those offering vision-related services.[20] Receipt of rehabilitation services can lead to a better quality of life, can increase the opportunity for an individual to become more social, and can increase the capacity to provide support to family and friends. As noted by Reinhardt, social support provision is a critical factor for adaptation and can increase life satisfaction.[21]

Research has shown that social support can positively affect health and health behavior in general.[22] However, minimal research has been carried out which explores the specific relationship between social support and depression in visually impaired individuals. Further research is therefore needed on how factors such as types of support and size of social network relate to adaptation, depression, and emotional distress.

DIRECTIONS FOR FUTURE RESEARCH

Patients like Lindy Bergman, who exhibit humor, a concern for others, a positive disposition, and a willingness to work hard at rehabilitative efforts, prompt questions about the link between attitude and level of visual function. While it is clear that psychosocial factors need to be addressed in the population of older people with visual impairment, the best method of doing so remains unclear. Age-related vision loss is a growing problem, and a concerted effort is needed to approach this issue strategically. Future research is an important component in the development of improvements in prevention and care, and the design of effective rehabilitation plans.

Research in the Low Vision Research Laboratory at The Chicago Lighthouse is focused on developing scientifically based strategies to help patients with visual impairment perform daily tasks in the most efficient manner. These strategies also encompass methods in which to gain a better understanding of the ways in which an individual is emotionally affected by vision loss and how it may affect treatment outcomes, and ways this knowledge may be utilized to determine the best method for intervention. The mission of the Low Vision Research Laboratory at The Chicago Lighthouse is to further formulate strategies for improving visual function and to learn more about treatment of mood, to develop better interventions for patients, and to disseminate findings to the community at large.

Factors that may contribute to better learning a new method of seeing and reading are positive attitude and a readiness to learn. Mrs. Bergman exhibited those character-istics in abundance, as well as an enthusiasm to do what-ever she could to improve her situation and to help benefit others as well. As indicated in Chapter 9, on the psychoso-cial and emotional reactions to vision loss, these character-istics may be related to an individual's effective use of low vision services. Investigating the factors that may influence more successful outcomes of low vision services is an im-portant direction for future research in the Low Vision Re-search Laboratory.

REFERENCES

1. Caroline C. Klaver, Roger C. Wolfs, Johannes R. Vingerling, Albert Hofman, and Paulus T. de Jong, "Age-Specific Prevalence and Causes of Blindness and Visual Impairment in an Older Population: The Rotterdam Study," *Archives of Ophthalmology* 116, no. 5 (1998): 653–58.

2. Jon S. Karlsson, "Self-Reports of Psychological Distress in Connection with Various Degrees of Visual Impairment," *Journal of Visual Impairment & Blindness* 92, no. 7 (1998): 483–90; Janet P. Szlyk, Jillian E. Becker, Gerald A. Fishman, and William Seiple, "Psycho-logical Profiles of Patients with Central Vision Loss," *Journal of Visual Impairment & Blindness* 94, no. 12 (2000): 781–90; Amy Horowitz, Joann P. Reinhardt, Kathrin Boerner, and Linda A. Travis, "The In-fluence of Health, Social Support Quality, and Rehabilitation on De-pression among Disabled Elders," *Aging & Mental Health* 7, no. 5 (2003): 342–50; Mark W. Bragg, "Vision Loss, Depression and Reha-bilitation," *International Congress Series* 1282 (Sept. 2005): 40–41; Gwyn Rees, Hui Wen Tee, Manjula Marella, Eva Fenwick, Mohamed Dirani, and Ecosse Lamoureux, "Vision-Specific Distress and Depres-sive Symptoms in People with Vision Impairment," *Investigative Oph-thalmology & Visual Science* 51, no. 6 (2010): 2891–96.

3. Bragg, "Vision Loss, Depression and Rehabilitation"; Rees et al., "Vision-Specific Distress and Depressive Symptoms"; Barbara L. Brody, Anthony C. Gamst, Rebecca A. Williams, Amanda R. Smith,

Phillip W. Lau, Douglas Dolnak, Mark H. Rapaport, Robert M. Kaplan, and Stuart I. Brown, "Depression, Visual Acuity, Comorbidity, and Disability Associated with Age-Related Macular Degeneration," *Ophthalmology* 108, no. 10 (2001): 1893–1901; Laura E. Dreer, Timothy R. Elliott, Jack Berry, Donald C. Fletcher, Marsha Swanson, and J. Christopher McNeal, "Cognitive Appraisals, Distress and Disability among Persons in Low Vision Rehabilitation," *British Journal of Health Psychology* 13, no. 3 (2008): 449–61; Nancy Groves, "Patients with AMD Benefit from Self-Management Training: Course Offers Lasting Effects with Patients Exhibiting Self-Confidence, Less Emotional Distress," *Ophthalmology Times,* Oct. 1, 2005, 32–33.

4. Barry W. Rovner, Robin J. Casten, and William S. Tasman, "Effect of Depression on Vision Function in Age-Related Macular Degeneration," *Archives of Ophthalmology* 120, no. 8 (2002): 1041–44; Barry W. Rovner and Mary Ganguli, "Depression and Disability Associated with Impaired Vision: The MoVies Project," *Journal of the American Geriatrics Society* 46, no. 5 (1998): 617–19; Barry W. Rovner, Pamela Zisselman, and Yocheved Shmuely-Dulitzki, "Depression and Disability in Elderly Persons with Impaired Vision: A Follow-Up Study," *Journal of the American Geriatrics Society* 44 (1996): 181–84; Patricia Grant, William Seiple, and Janet Szlyk, "The Impact of Depression on the Actual and Perceived Effects of Vision Rehabilitation," *Journal of Rehabilitation Research and Development* 48, no. 9 (2011).

5. Rovner and Ganguli, "Depression and Disability Associated with Impaired Vision."

6. Rovner et al., "Depression and Disability in Elderly Persons"; Grant et al., "The Impact of Depression"; Cynthia Owsley, Gerald McGwin, Paul P. Lee, Nicole Wasserman, and Karen Searcey, "Characteristics of Low-Vision Rehabilitation Services in the United States," *Archives of Ophthalmology* 127, no. 5 (2009): 681–89.

7. Bragg, "Vision Loss, Depression and Rehabilitation."

8. Owsley et al., "Characteristics of Low-Vision Rehabilitation Services."

9. Grant et al., "The Impact of Depression."

10. Horowitz et al., "Influence of Health, Social Support Quality, and Rehabilitation."

11. Amy Horowitz, Joann P. Reinhardt, and Kathrin Boerner, "The Effect of Rehabilitation on Depression among Visually Impaired Older Adults," *Aging & Mental Health* 9 (2005): 563–70.

12. Rees et al., "Vision-Specific Distress and Depressive Symptoms."

13. Rebecca A. Williams, Barbara L. Brody, Ronald G. Thomas, Robert M. Kaplan, and Stuart I. Brown, "The Psychosocial Impact of Macular Degeneration," *Archives of Ophthalmology* 116, no. 4 (1998): 514–20.

14. Dreer et al., "Cognitive Appraisals, Distress and Disability."

15. Karen Glanz, Barbara K. Rimer, and Frances Marcus Lewis, *Health Behavior and Health Education: Theory, Research and Practice* (San Francisco: Wiley & Sons, 2002).

16. Kathrin Boerner, Joann P. Reinhardt, and Amy Horowitz, "The Effect of Rehabilitation Service Use on Coping Patterns over Time among Older Adults with Age-Related Vision Loss," *Clinical Rehabilitation* 20, no. 6 (2006): 478–87.

17. Richard S. Lazarus and Susan Folkman, *Stress, Appraisal and Coping* (New York: Springer, 1984).

18. Joann P. Reinhardt, "Effects of Positive and Negative Support Received and Provided on Adaptation to Chronic Visual Impairment," *Applied Developmental Science* 5, no. 2 (2001): 76–85.

19. Horowitz et al., "Influence of Health, Social Support Quality, and Rehabilitation."

20. Reinhardt, "Effects of Positive and Negative Support."

21. Ibid.

22. Catherine A. Heaney and Barbara Israel, "Social Networks and Social Support," in *Health Behavior and Health Education: Theory, Research, and Practice,* ed. K. Glanz, B. Rimer, and F. M. Lewis, 3rd ed., 185–209 (San Francisco: Jossey-Bass, 2002).

Appendix
Age-Related Macular Degeneration Guide

A ge-related macular degeneration (AMD) is occurring at a rapid rate in this country. According to the American Academy of Ophthalmology (AAO), 10 to 15 million individuals have the condition and about 10 percent of those affected have the wet type of AMD ("Are You at Risk," 2010).

RISK FACTORS

According to the AAO, if you have at least two of the top-five risk factors listed below, you should consider having an eye examination by an ophthalmologist or other medical eye specialist and learn what you can do to reduce your risks (AAO, 2010).

+ Smoking
+ Obesity
+ Age (Over 60 Years Old)
+ Hypertension
+ Family History of AMD

Source: Adapted from "Macular Degeneration Guide," Senior Site, American Foundation for the Blind, www.afb.org.

Smoking

Current smokers have a two-to-three times higher risk for developing AMD than people who have never smoked. Quitting smoking can reduce your risk of developing AMD (Thornton et al., 2005). (See Chapter 3 for additional discussion.)

Obesity

Being obese doubles the risk of developing advanced macular degeneration (van Leeuwen et al., 2003). Losing weight via a healthy diet and regular exercise can reduce your risk of developing AMD. For more information, see the "Ways to Reduce Your Risk" section in this article.

Age (Over 60 Years Old)

Although AMD may occur earlier, studies indicate that people over age 60 are at greater risk than those in younger age groups. For instance, a large study found that people in middle age have about a 2 percent risk of getting AMD, but this risk increased to nearly 30 percent in those over age 75 (NEI, 2009). (See also Chapters 7 and 8.)

Hypertension

The National Eye Institute's (NEI) Age-Related Eye Disease Study indicated that persons with hypertension were 1.5 times as likely to develop wet macular degeneration compared with persons without hypertension (NEI, 2009).

Family History of AMD

Studies indicate that having a parent, child, or sibling with macular degeneration can mean your chances of developing the condition are 2.5 times higher than people with no close relatives with AMD (Fine, Berger, Maguire, & Ho, 2000). Further, your lifetime risk for developing AMD can be up to four times higher if you have close relatives with the condition. While not all AMD is hereditary, certain genes have been strongly associated with a person's risk of AMD, and genetic predisposition may account for half the cases of AMD in this country (Haines et al., 2005).

Other Possible Risk Factors

+ **Gender.** Women appear to be more at risk of AMD than men (NEI, 2009).
+ **Race.** Whites are much more likely to lose vision from AMD than African Americans (NEI, 2009).
+ **Exposure to Sunlight.** Exposure to higher energy (blue) light waves may damage the macula. This exposure can be limited by sunglasses that have a yellow tint, which blocks blue light waves. In addition, eating green and leafy vegetables may be of benefit in forming macular pigment that can absorb blue light waves. See the "Ways to Reduce Your Risk" section in this article for more dietary guidance.
+ **Heart Disease.** Macular degeneration is also linked to coronary heart disease (AAO, 2009).

WAYS TO REDUCE YOUR RISK

Get Moving

Incorporate exercise into your every day life. (See Chapter 3 for additional discussion.)

Eat Healthfully

Dr. Lylas Mogk (2003), noted ophthalmologist and author on macular degeneration, offers the following suggestions (see Chapter 3 for additional discussion):

1. Eat an abundance of dark green leafy vegetables like kale, collard greens, and spinach. These types of vegetables contain a lot of lutein, which protects the macula from sun damage, just as it protects the leaves from sun damage.
2. Eat fatty fish regularly. These types of fish are high in omega-3 fatty acids, which help decrease inflammation and promote eye health.
3. Avoid packaged foods as much as possible. It's important to keep a balance between omega-6 fatty acids and omega-3 fatty acids in our diets. Virtually every food in a package contains omega-6 fatty acids in the form of vegetable oil. We need to increase our intake of omega-3s and decrease our intake of omega-6s.
4. Avoid artificial fats. Low-fat foods are good options if they've achieved their low-fat status through a process that physically removes the fat. Skim milk and low fat cottage cheese are examples of these types of low-fat foods. A low-fat cookie or a no-fat cake, however, is a nutritional oxymoron; that is, usually a low-fat or no-fat label on baked goods doesn't mean less fat was used in the production of the food, but that an artificial fat was used, usually partially hydrogenated vegetable oil. These types of fats are artificial ingredients made in a laboratory and our bodies can't metabolize them. So, it's best to eat real cookies—just don't eat the whole dozen!

Stop Smoking

Stopping smoking can reduce your risk of developing AMD.

Lower Blood Pressure and Lose Weight

Follow your doctor's orders.

Schedule Regular Eye Evaluations

If you have not had an eye exam by an ophthalmologist in three or more years, you may qualify for help from the AMD Eye Care Program offered through the AAO. The program provides free eye exams for individuals who have not been diagnosed with AMD, are age 65 and older, are U.S. citizens or legal residents, and do not belong to an HMO or the VA. Call the toll-free helpline at 1-866-324-EYES (3937) for more information. (See also Chapters 3 and 10.)

QUESTIONS TO ASK YOUR DOCTOR

If you have been diagnosed with AMD, or are expecting a diagnosis of AMD, you may feel overwhelmed and unsure of what to ask when you visit your doctor for your exam. The list of questions below was developed by an ophthalmologist. The next time you visit your doctor, you may want to bring this list with you for guidance and ask all or many of the following questions:

+ What is the diagnosis?
+ What tests were used to make this diagnosis?
+ What caused the condition?
+ Is it hereditary? Do I need to get my relatives checked?
+ Are there any symptoms or changes I should watch for?
+ What kind of eye care professional(s) (ophthalmologist, subspecialist, optometrist, low vision specialist) would be best to monitor/treat my condition?
+ Which kind of eye care professional are you? Are you a medical doctor?
+ How often should I see you or any other eye specialist?
+ Can my condition be treated?

✦ What are the preferred treatments for my condition? Laser surgery? Medications or vitamins? Injections?

✦ What are the risks/benefits/alternatives for these treatments and what is the recovery period?

✦ Will anesthesia be used for any of these treatments? What type?

✦ When should the treatment start and how long will it last?

✦ Will there be any pain or discomfort associated with my treatment? If so, how long will it last?

✦ How often do you anticipate that I will need to return for follow up to monitor the treatment?

✦ Are there food/drugs/activities I should avoid while undergoing this treatment?

✦ What kind of tests are involved for ongoing care and how often will I need them?

✦ What do you expect to find out from these tests?

✦ When will we know the results and can you explain them?

✦ Do I have to do anything special to prepare for these tests?

✦ Do the tests carry any risks or side effects?

✦ Will you send the test results to my primary care physician?

✦ Are there things I can do to monitor my own eye condition? I have heard of the Amsler grid. Should I use one?

✦ What happens if my treatments do not help enough and I still have vision problems?

✦ Should I begin making any lifestyle changes such as exercise, diet, cessation of smoking, routine daily living?

✦ Are there services or products that will help, such as magnification, special devices, or services for people experiencing vision loss? (For information on services for people with vision loss, see the *AFB Directory of Services,* available at www.afb.org.)

(See Chapter 10 for a detailed discussion of the low vision eye exam.)

TREATMENTS

Treatments differ for the wet and dry types of macular degeneration; new research is ongoing. (See Chapter 8 in this book for more information.)

TIPS FOR LIVING WITH MACULAR DEGENERATION

Macular degeneration may affect your vision as follows:

+ Diminished ability to see detail, such as text and faces
+ Presence of a spot or "scotoma" near the center of vision, and/or distortion, blurriness, and waviness in lines, text, and faces
+ Reduction in light; things appear darker
+ Diminished ability to see things that are in poor contrast

Despite these challenges, you can continue to successfully manage your everyday tasks. See the Resources listed following this appendix, the chapters in this book, and www .afb.org for more information. In addition, the following two suggestions may be beneficial:

Eccentric Viewing

AMD affects central vision the most. To help you minimize the impact of the blind spot or distortion that you may have near the center of your vision, practice eccentric viewing by learning to look slightly to the side (or up or down). When viewing your TV screen, dinner plate, or reading material, imagine that you are looking at a clock face. While focusing at the center of the monitor, plate, or text, look to the right toward 3 o'clock, then to the left toward 9 o'clock, and so on through the positions of the numbers on the clock face. Determine which clock position helps you see items in the center of your field of vision better. You may also try moving your dinner plate or reading materials to the side (the same clock position that you found most helpful to look toward), in order to see them better. By moving the object slightly to the side (or up or down), your eyes will follow, and you will see "around" the distortion or blind spot more easily, and probably more clearly, than if you look straight down. (See Chapter 10 for additional information.)

Improved Lighting

Due to macular degeneration, objects may appear darker, mainly because of damage to the cone cells on your retina, which receive and process light. Try using an inexpensive gooseneck lamp, available at many stores for about $15, to provide extra light on the desk or table where you eat, write, read, and do other tasks. Position the lamp close to you and to the side. When you need to plug something in or turn a key, use a bright flashlight (such as the new LED flashlights) to shine more light on your task. Purchase a few press-on battery operated lamps to attach to the wall of a closet to help you pick out your clothes, or apply them to the inside of your cupboards to help you see your dishes.

An LED press-on lamp, while slightly more expensive than the older, incandescent models, will last much longer (often several years) and be much brighter.

Improved lighting and slight eccentric viewing can make a considerable difference in how well you see.

Employing these strategies may help you to successfully perform the tasks that you want to do.

REFERENCES

American Academy of Ophthalmology. "Are You at Risk for Age-Related Macular Degeneration (AMD)? Learn the Top 5 Risk Factors." 2010, www.aao.org/newsroom/release/20100303.cfm.

———. "Positive Trend Found for Diabetic Eye Health; Macular Degeneration Linked to Heart Disease; How Poor Vision Impacts Social, Economic Success." 2009, www.aao.org/newsroom/release/20091001.cfm.

Fine, S. L., J. W. Berger, M. G. Maquire, and A. C. Ho. "Age-Related Macular Degeneration." *New England Journal of Medicine* 342, no. 7 (2000): 483–91.

Haines, J. L., M. A. Hauser, S. Schmidt, W. K. Scott, L. M. Olson, P. Gallins, K. L. Spencer, S. Y. Kwan, M. Noureddine, J. R. Gilbert, N. Schnetz-Boutaud, A. Agarwal, E. A. Postel, and M. A. Pericak-Vance. "Complement Factor H Variant Increases the Risk of Age-Related Macular Degeneration." *Science* 308, no. 5720 (2005): 419–21. doi:10.1126/science.1110359.

Mogk, L., and M. Mogk. *Macular Degeneration: The Complete Guide to Saving Your Sight.* New York: Ballantine Books, 2003.

National Eye Institute. "Facts About Age-Related Macular Degeneration." 2009, www.nei.nih.gov/health/maculardegen/armd_facts.asp.

Thornton, J., R. Edwards, P. Mitchell, R. A. Harrison, I. Buchan, and S. P. Kelly. "Smoking and Age-Related Macular Degeneration: A Review of Association." *Eye* 19, no. 9 (2005): 935–44.

van Leeuwen, R., C. C. W. Klaver, J. R. Vingerling, A. Hofman, and P. T. V. M. de Jong. "The Risk and Natural Course of Age-Related Maculopathy: Follow-up at 6½ Years in the Rotterdam Study." *Archives of Ophthalmology* 121 (April 2003): 519–26.

RESOURCES

Duffy, M., *Making Life More Livable.* New York: AFB Press, 2002.

Orr, A., and P. Rogers. *Aging and Vision Loss: A Handbook for Families.* New York: AFB Press, 2006.

Reingold, N. *Out of the Corner of My Eye.* New York: AFB Press, 2007.

Roberts, D. L. *The First Year: Age-Related Macular Degeneration: An Essential Guide for the Newly Diagnosed.* New York: Marlowe & Company, 2006.

Resources

This resource listing provides a sample of the organizations and companies that offer assistance, information, referrals, products, and services related to vision loss and aging for both professionals and individuals who have visual impairment and their families. The listings include national organizations that are sources of general information on vision loss; organizations that focus specifically on macular degeneration or other vision conditions commonly experienced by older people; reading resources that provide Talking Books and other access to reading materials for people with vision loss; and sources of products for independent living.

These listings provide only a representative sample of the resources available in these areas. A comprehensive list of service providers may be found in the *AFB Directory of Services for Blind and Visually Impaired Persons in the United States and Canada,* available from the American Foundation for the Blind website at www .afb.org.

American Foundation for the Blind
2 Penn Plaza, Suite 1102
New York, NY 10121
(800) 232-5463 (800-AFB-LINE) or (212) 502-7600
Fax: (212) 502-7777
E-mail: afbinfo@afb.net
www.afb.org

National organization and information clearinghouse for people who are visually impaired, their families, the public, professionals, schools, organizations, and corporations; it provides wide-ranging web-based and published resources, undertakes professional development and training programs, and operates a toll-free information hotline. Provides consultative services, conducts research, and mounts program initiatives to promote accessibility and the inclusion of visually impaired persons in society and employment; advocates for services, legislation, and access to information and products; and maintains the Helen Keller Archives. Publishes books, electronic products, DVDs, the *AFB Directory of Services for Blind and Visually Impaired Persons in the United States and Canada*, the *Journal of Visual Impairment & Blindness,* and *AccessWorld: Technology and People with Visual Impairments.* Maintains CareerConnect (www.Career Connect.org), a website on the range and diversity of jobs performed by adults who are blind or visually impaired throughout the United States and Canada that offers job-seeking resources to visually impaired persons and information to employers; FamilyConnect (www .FamilyConnect.org), a website for families of children with visual impairments; and SeniorSite (www.afb.org/SeniorSite), a website that connects seniors, family members, and caregivers to local services and showcases a wide range of assisted living products available to people with vision loss. In addition to its New York City headquarters and Public Policy Center in Washington, D.C., AFB maintains offices in Atlanta, Dallas, and Huntington, West Virginia.

The Chicago Lighthouse for People Who Are Blind or Visually Impaired

1850 West Roosevelt Road
Chicago, IL 60608
(312) 666-1331
Fax: (312) 243-8539
TDD/TTY: (312) 666-8874
www.thechicagolighthouse.org

One of the nation's most comprehensive social service agencies offering nearly 30 programs and services for people who are blind or visually impaired, including educational, clinical, vocational, and rehabilitation services for children, youths, and adults who are blind or visually impaired, including people who are deaf-blind and multiply disabled. Programs include Bergman Institute for Psychological Support; Sandy and Rick Forsythe Center for Comprehensive Vision Care; Pangere Center for Inherited Retinal Diseases; the Dr. Alfred A. Rosenbloom Low Vision Rehabilitation Service (which includes a network of satellite locations around Chicago and suburbs); the Adaptive Technology Center; and the Low Vision Research Laboratory, as well as a range of programs in education, employment, and independent living. The Lighthouse also houses CRIS Radio (Chicagoland Radio Information Service), which broadcasts news, entertainment, and sports to people who cannot read due to visual impairments or other disabilities; the Kane Legal Clinic, which helps people who are visually impaired with legal problems at no charge; and the Instructional Materials Center for the State of Illinois. The Lighthouse's independent living program offers daily living skills training to adults who are blind, as well as prevocational training, individual and group counseling, recreation and leisure activities, and assistance with daily living. Also provides social services, crisis intervention, functional assessment, advocacy, and appropriate referrals for deaf-blind persons in the community and in other programs, and a broad range of instructional and social activities for seniors. Also houses the Tools for Living Retail Store, which offers a wide range of products for people who are blind or visually impaired.

NATIONAL ORGANIZATIONS

American Academy of Ophthalmology
655 Beach Street
San Francisco, CA 94109
(415) 561-8500
Fax: (415) 561-8533
E-mail: customer_service@aao.org
www.aao.org

National membership association of ophthalmologists that offers print and electronic educational materials, including reference books, audiotapes, videotapes, CDs, self-assessment programs, and an online education center. Sponsors Eye Care America to give free eye care to elderly persons (see separate listing).

American Council of the Blind
2200 Wilson Boulevard, Suite 650
Arlington, VA 22201
(800) 424-8666 or (202) 467-5081
Fax: (703) 465-5085
E-mail: info@acb.org
www.acb.org

National consumer organization that serves as a national clearinghouse for information and promotes the effective participation of blind people in all aspects of society. Provides information and referral; legal assistance and representation; scholarships; leadership and legislative training; consumer advocate support; assistance in technological research; a speaker referral service; consultative and advisory services to individuals, organizations, and agencies; and assistance with developing programs. Interest groups include the Alliance on Aging and Vision Loss and the Council of Citizens with Low Vision International. Publishes the *Braille Forum.*

American Diabetes Association
1701 North Beauregard Street
Alexandria, VA 22314
(800) 342-2383
E-mail: AskADA@diabetes.org
www.diabetes.org

National membership organization that provides information and public education about diabetes, including diabetic retinopathy, to consumers and professionals. Publishes books, journals, and brochures and funds research to prevent, cure, and manage diabetes.

American Optometric Association
243 North Lindbergh Boulevard
St. Louis, MO 63141
(314) 991-4100
Fax: (314) 991-4101
www.aoanet.org
www.aoa.org/visionusa.xml

Federation of state, student, and armed forces optometric associations working to provide the public with quality vision and eye care. Sets professional standards, lobbies government and other organizations on behalf of the optometric profession, and provides research and education leadership. Sponsors VISION USA, a program developed by its members to provide basic eye health and vision care services free of charge to uninsured, low-income people and their families (see separate listing).

Bioptic Driving Network
5520 Ridgeton Hill Court
Fairfax, VA 22032
(413) 638-6941
http://biopticdriving.org

Voluntary organization that serves the needs and interests of those with stable low vision who may be able to drive with a bioptic telescope system, by providing technical and experiential information about it.

Blinded Veterans Association
477 H Street, NW
Washington, DC 20001-2694
(202) 371-8880
Fax: (202) 371-8258
E-mail: bva@bva.org
www.bva.org

Provides support and assistance to blind veterans to enable them to take advantage of rehabilitation and vocational training benefits, job placement services, and other aid from federal, state, and local resources.

Eldercare Locator
U.S. Administration on Aging
Washington, DC 20201
(800) 677-1116
E-mail: eldercarelocator@n4a.org
www.eldercare.gov

A public service of the U.S. Administration on Aging that connects older Americans and their caregivers with sources of information on senior services and links those who need assistance with state and local area agencies on aging and community-based organizations that serve older adults and their caregivers.

Eye Care America
P.O. Box 429098
San Francisco, CA 94142-9098
(800) 222-3937 or (887) 888-6327
Fax: (415) 561-8567
www.eyecareamerica.org

A public service foundation of the American Academy of Ophthalmology that provides eye examinations and up to one year of care to U.S. citizens and legal residents through a network of volunteer ophthalmologists around the country, often at no out-of-pocket cost to those who qualify.

Foundation Fighting Blindness
7168 Columbia Gateway Drive, Suite 100
Columbia, MD 21046
(800) 683-5555 or (410) 423-0600
TDD: (800) 683-5551
E-mail: info@fightblindness.org
www.blindness.org

Organization supporting research on the cause, prevention, and treatment for people affected by retinitis pigmentosa (RP), macular degeneration, Usher syndrome, and the entire spectrum of retinal degenerative diseases. Holds regional and national workshops for volunteers and professionals.

Lighthouse International
111 East 59th Street
New York, NY 10022-1202
(800) 829-0500 or (212) 821-9200
Fax: (212) 821-0707
TTD/TTY: (212) 821-9713

E-mail: info@lighthouse.org
www.lighthouse.org

National clearinghouse on vision impairment and vision rehabilitation. Provides low vision and rehabilitation services, including training in adaptive living skills and computer skills for seniors. Maintains a catalog and an online store of independent living products.

National Eye Institute
Building 31, Room 6A32
31 Center Drive, MSC 2510
Bethesda, MD 20892-2510
(301) 496-5248
Fax: (301) 402-1065
E-mail: 2020@nei.nih.gov
www.nei.nih.gov

U.S. federal agency established by Congress in 1968 to protect and prolong the vision of the American people. Conducts and supports research that helps prevent and treat eye diseases and other disorders of vision. Provides information on advances in eye disease research and about clinical trials.

National Federation of the Blind
200 East Wells Street at Jernigan Place
Baltimore, MD 21230
(410) 659-9314
Fax: (410) 685-5653
E-mail: nfb@nfb.org
www.nfb.org

National consumer organization that works to improve the social and economic conditions of people who are blind. Monitors legislation affecting blind people, assists in promoting needed services, provides evaluation of present programs and assistance in establishing new ones, grants scholarships, and conducts a public education program. Publishes the *Braille Monitor* and *Future Reflections*.

Prevent Blindness America
211 West Wacker Drive, Suite 1700
Chicago, IL 60606
(800) 331-2020
www.preventblindness.org/about-us

Volunteer eye health and safety organization dedicated to fighting blindness and saving sight. Conducts a program of public and professional education, research, and industrial and community services to prevent blindness. Its services include promotion of local glaucoma screening programs, vision testing, and eye safety, and dissemination of information on low vision devices and clinics. Maintains a network of state affiliates.

U.S. Department of Veterans Affairs Blind Rehabilitation Service
810 Vermont Avenue, NW
Washington, DC 20420
(800) 827-1000
www.va.gov/blindrehab

U.S. federal agency that oversees services for visually impaired veterans through a network of rehabilitation centers, clinics, and field staff throughout the country. Services include orientation and mobility, living skills, communication skills, activities of daily living, manual skills, computer access training, physical conditioning, recreation, adjustment to blindness, family counseling, and group meetings. Also supplies needed devices, appliances, and equipment.

VISION USA
243 North Lindbergh Boulevard
St. Louis, MO 63141
(800) 766-4466
Fax: (314) 991-4101
E-mail: visionusa@aoa.org
www.aoa.org/visionusa.xml

Program of the American Optometric Association to provide basic eye health and vision care services free of charge to uninsured, low-income people and their families.

ORGANIZATIONS FOR MACULAR DEGENERATION AND OTHER EYE CONDITIONS

American Retina Foundation
6816 Southpoint Parkway, Suite 1000
Jacksonville, FL 32216
(904) 998-0356
www.americanretina.org
www.savingvision.org

Organization formed by the American Society of Retina Specialists (ASRS) to promote public awareness, continuing medical education, research, and treatment of retinal diseases. Developed www.savingvision.org, an online web project that features an interactive slide presentation, brochure, and patient resources concerning age-related macular degeneration and other retinal diseases.

American Society of Cataract and Refractive Surgery
4000 Legato Road, Suite 700
Fairfax, VA 22033
(703) 591-2220
Fax: (703) 591-0614
E-mail: ascrs@ascrs.org
www.ascrs.org

Membership organization that provides information about cataracts and refractive surgery and referrals to ophthalmologists specializing in eye surgery. Publishes the *Journal of Cataract & Refractive Surgery, Eye World Magazine,* and *EyeWorld News Service.*

American Society of Retina Specialists
20 North Wacker Drive, Suite 2234
Chicago, IL 60606
(312) 578-8760
www.asrs.org

Professional organization of vitreoretinal specialists. Provides referrals to retinal specialists all over the world through its website. Promote public awareness, continuing medical education, research, and treatment of retinal diseases through its charitable arm, the American Retina Foundation.

Association for Macular Diseases
210 East 64th Street
New York, NY 10021
(800) 365-2219 or (212) 605-3719
Fax: (212) 606-3795
E-mail: association@retinal-research.org
http://macula.org/about-us

Nationwide support group for individuals with macular degeneration and their families. Provides resources and assistance while promoting research and education.

Glaucoma Foundation
80 Maiden Lane, Suite 700
New York, NY 10038
(212) 285-0080
E-mail: info@glaucomafoundation.org
www.glaucomafoundation.org

Research organization dedicated to eradicating blindness from glaucoma through vital research and public education. Serves patients nationally and internationally through its website, online support groups, and local chapters in Greater Chicago, Long Island (New York), New England, and New York City. Offers free glaucoma screenings, funds research, and publishes consumer guides and brochures and *Eye to Eye*, a quarterly newsletter.

Macular Degeneration Foundation
P.O. Box 531313
Henderson, NV 89053
(888) 633-3937
Fax: (702) 450-3396
E-mail: eyesight@eyesight.org
www.eyesight.org

Medical research and educational foundation that supports research to inhibit the progression of macular degeneration and restore vision. Publishes *The Magnifier* newsletter.

Macular Degeneration International
(800) 683-5555
E-mail: MDInfo@blindness.org
www.maculardegeneration.org

Support organization for the Foundation Fighting Blindness to help patients with macular degeneration live independent and productive lives.

Macular Degeneration Partnership
6222 Wilshire Boulevard, Suite 260
Los Angeles, CA 90048
(310) 623-4466
Fax: (310) 623-1937
E-mail: ContactUs@AMD.org
www.AMD.org

Coalition of patients and families, researchers, clinicians, industry partners, and leaders in the fields of vision and aging, collaborating to disseminate information about age-related macular degeneration, provide support to patients, and marshal resources for a cure. Maintains a Help Center on the Internet that provides users with links to websites for health, aging, and low vision information, along with tools and other related resources.

Macular Degeneration Support Group
3600 Blue Ridge Boulevard
Grandview, MO 64030
(816) 761-7080
E-mail: director@mdsupport.org
www.mdsupport.org

Online support group for people affected by macular degeneration and similar retinal diseases. Offers a public awareness program designed to reach people who are without Internet access.

RESOURCES FOR READING

Audible.com
One Washington Park
Newark, NJ 07102
(888) 283-5051 or 973-820-0400
www.audible.com

Commercial online source of audio books, magazines, newspapers, and programs that can be downloaded from the Internet and listened to on an MP3 player, a computer, or a mobile device or copied to a CD and listened to on a CD player.

Books Aloud
150 East San Fernando Street
San Jose, CA 95112-3580
(408) 808-2613
Fax: (408) 808-4625
E-mail: info@booksaloud.org
www.booksaloud.org

Audio library that offers "Reading by Listening" program, which provides a wide variety of recorded reading material free of charge on standard cassettes or CDs to eligible individuals.

Bookshare.org
Benetech
480 South California Avenue
Palo Alto, CA 94306
Phone: (650) 352-0198
Fax: (650) 475-1066
www.bookshare.org

Free online library for individuals with a print disability. Books can be downloaded from the Internet and read aloud with free software or read with braille-reading equipment.

Choice Magazine Listening
85 Channel Drive
Port Washington, NY 11050
(888) 724-6423 or (516) 883-8280

Fax: (516) 944-6849

E-mail: choicemag@aol.com

www.choicemagazinelistening.org

Free monthly anthology of current articles chosen from over 100 leading magazines recorded in four-track Library of Congress format and distributed for free through regional libraries. Also available to download, free of charge, onto a computer through the National Library Service for the Blind and Physically Handicapped, Library of Congress (NLS) (https://nls.loc.gov). Digital Talking Book machines required to listen to the downloaded material are available from NLS.

International Association of Audio Information Services

(800) 280-5325

Fax: (504) 776-2727

www.iaais.org

International organization of radio reading services, which provides audio access to information for people who are print disabled (blind, visually impaired, learning disabled, or physically disabled), including news, feature stories, sports, advertisements, and other special programs. Connects listeners with services in their area. Provides a comprehensive list of all member audio information services on its website at www.iaais.org/findservices.html.

Matilda Ziegler Magazine

e-mail: editor@matildaziegler.com

www.matildaziegler.com

Online magazine that features general interest news and blindness-related information.

National Library Service for the Blind and Physically Handicapped

Library of Congress

1291 Taylor Street, NW

Washington, DC 20542

(800) 424-8567 or (202) 707-5100

Fax: (202) 707-0712

TDD/TTY: (202) 707-0744

E-mail: nls@loc.gov
www.loc.gov/nls

Free library service for people who are unable to read standard print materials because of a visual or physical impairment. Provides recorded Talking Books and magazines on cassette or digital cartridge and braille publications to eligible borrowers by postage-free mail and through a network of cooperative libraries. Also distributes Talking Book machines.

SOURCES OF INDEPENDENT LIVING PRODUCTS

The companies listed in this section sell a wide variety of specialized products that help people with visual impairments and other disabilities carry out everyday activities.

Ableware/Maddak
6 Industrial Road
Pequannock, NJ 07440
(800) 443-4926 or (973) 628-7600
Fax: (973) 305-0841
E-mail: custservice@maddak.com
www.maddak.com

Designs and manufactures assistive devices for activities of daily living. Specializes in home healthcare and rehabilitation products for the senior, disability, and rehabilitation markets. Offers adapted games, adapted scissors, eating utensils and tableware, enlarged grips, nonskid table mats, and writing devices.

Adaptive Solutions
1301 Azalea Road, Suite 102
Mobile, AL 33619-1087
(800) 299-3045 or (251) 666-3045
E-mail: Fax: (251) 660-1788
www.talksight.com

Distributes a variety of assistive technology products for people who are blind and visually impaired. Also offers training programs for software and hardware products.

AdaptiveVoice LLC
25286 Adelanto
Laguna Niguel, CA 92677
(949) 436-7760
Fax: (949) 419-3506
E-mail: Randyce@AdaptiveVoice.com
www.adaptivevoice.com/

Distributes CDesk, a program that enables people with visual impairments to perform multiple functions on a computer with minimal training.

American Printing House for the Blind
1839 Frankfort Avenue
P.O. Box 6085
Louisville, KY 40206-0085
(800) 223-1839 or (502) 895-2405
Fax: (502) 899-2274
E-mail: info@aph.org
www.aph.org

Creates and distributes braille products, books, and supplies; large-print books; computer software and access products; labeling and marking products; lighting; low vision devices; mobility devices; personal care products; recreation and leisure products; talking products; and writing and reading devices.

The Chicago Lighthouse for People Who Are Blind or Visually Impaired Tools for Living Retail Store
1850 West Roosevelt Road
Chicago, IL 60608
(800) 919-3375 or (312) 997-3683
Fax: (312) 506-0110
E-mail: store@chicagolighthouse.org
www.chicagolighthouse.org/store

Offers a wide range of unique products for people who are blind or visually impaired to assist them to be independent in their daily lives, including but not limited to large-button telephones and cell phones; kitchen items and independent living aids; sunglasses; white canes; portable and magnifying lamps; portable, handheld, and video magnifiers (CCTVs); and accessibility software and computer aids.

Clotilde

P.O. Box 7500
Big Sandy, TX 75755-7500
(800) 545-4002
www.clotilde.com

Sells sewing notions, needle threaders, and regular and adaptive sewing supplies.

Dazor Manufacturing Corporation

2079 Congressional
St. Louis, MO 63146
(800) 345-9103 or (314) 652-2400
Fax: (314) 652-2069
E-mail: info@dazor.com
www.dazor.com

Manufactures a wide variety of task lights and lamps, including swing arm, combination fluorescent/incandescent, halogen, and magnifying lamps.

En-Vision America

1845 West Hovey Avenue
Normal, IL 61761
(800) 890-1180 or (309) 452-3088
Fax: (309) 452-3643
www.envisionamerica.com

Distributes ScripTalk, a portable, handheld audio system that reads prescriptions aloud.

Independent Living Aids

200 Robbins Lane
Jericho, NY 11753
(800) 537-2118 or (516) 937-1848
Fax: (516) 937-3906
E-mail: can-do@independentliving.com
www.independentliving.com

Distributes braille products and supplies, adapted clocks and watches, computer software and access products, diabetes management products, kitchen and housekeeping items, labeling and marking products, lighting, low vision devices, mobility devices, personal care products, recreation and leisure products, talking products, telephones and accessories, and writing and reading devices.

LS&S Group

P.O. Box 673
Northbrook, IL 60065
(800) 468-4789 or (716) 348-3500
Fax: (716) 873-3848
E-mail: info@lssproducts.com
www.lssproducts.com

Distributes braille products and supplies, adapted clocks and watches, computer software and access products, diabetes management products, kitchen and housekeeping items, labeling and marking products, lighting, low vision devices, mobility devices, personal care products, recreation and leisure products, talking products, telephones and accessories, and writing and reading devices.

Maxi-Aids

42 Executive Boulevard
Farmingdale, NY 11735
(800) 522-6294 or (631) 752-0521
Fax: (631) 752-0689
TTY: (631) 752-0738
www.maxiaids.com

Distributes braille products and supplies, adapted clocks and watches, computer software and access products, diabetes management products, kitchen and housekeeping items, labeling and marking products, lighting, low vision devices, mobility devices, personal care products, recreation and leisure products, talking products, telephones and accessories, and writing and reading devices.

Index